LIVING *with*
METASTATIC
BREAST CANCER

LIVING *with* METASTATIC BREAST CANCER

Stories of Faith and Hope

Charles L. Vogel MD, FACP

Breast Medical Oncologist
Baptist Health Miami Cancer Institute, Plantation, FL

Laura M. Freedman, MD

Associate Professor of Radiation Oncology
Sylvester Comprehensive Cancer Center
Miller School of Medicine
University of Miami

To order additional copies of this book, contact:
Xlibris
844-714-8691
www.Xlibris.com
Orders@Xlibris.com
835030

CONTENTS

To my wife, Patricia Vogel (née O'Toole), one of the strongest and most resilient women I have known. Survivor of four near-death experiences (none were breast cancer related), she looks twenty years younger than her stated age and is a devoted wife and doting grandmother to Mia, Jace, Benjamin, Max, and Bennett.

CHAPTER I

Introduction

This is a book about metastatic breast cancer (MBC) patients and intended for MBC patients. Newly diagnosed MBC patients are often told of the poor prognosis by their physician. In this internet age, this air of pessimism is reinforced, hence the need for a more optimistic counterbalance. This book was specifically written to provide this counterbalance. Doctors and publications deal largely with statistics, yet no individual is a statistic, and many exceptions to the norm exist. This book is about these exceptional patients and aims to serve as an inspiration to newly diagnosed patients with MBC who are looking for a ray of hope after receiving a diagnosis, which, at that moment, seems so devastating.

Most of these patients have been told by their physicians that MBC is considered as "essentially incurable." This statement is supported by a study out of MD Anderson Cancer Center where 1,500 newly diagnosed patients with MBC were treated initially with an aggressive chemotherapy regimen and then followed for fifteen years. At that point in time, regardless of intervening therapies, only 2.5% were still alive (1).

Although "essentially incurable" may well be correct, the phrase does *not* mean untreatable, and this book presents the clinical histories and personal stories of patients with MBC living long and productive lives.

While the stories of patients detailed here largely come from one oncologic practice, every oncologist in any practice has many such patients who should serve as an inspiration for others starting their own personal journey.

Before discussing MBC, a brief dialogue regarding breast cancer statistics is provided. This is to give important background information about the enormity of the problem and also to reemphasize to the reader that this book is a reminder that *you are not a statistic.*

In the latest compilation of cancer statistics, the estimated number of new breast cancer patients for 2020 is estimated to be 279,100, of which 276,480 are women and 2,620 are men. The estimated death rates for 2020 are 42,690, with 42,170 women and 520 men (2). In addition to this number, another 60,000 patients are diagnosed with ductal carcinoma in situ (considered stage 0 breast cancer) every year for which twenty-year cure rates are 97% in two large series from Canada (3) and the Netherlands (4).

Breast cancer is the most common cancer among women and the second most common cause of cancer deaths after lung cancer. Although it is highly publicized that one in eight women will develop breast cancer, that number includes the time frame from birth to death. In actuality, the numbers are more reassuring when broken down by age cohorts as seen in the table below.

Age	Birth to 49	50–59	60–69	>70
Risk	1 in 49	1 in 42	1 in 28	1 in 14

When one looks at the numbers based on stage from 2009 to 2015, the five-year overall survival rate is 90% but is up to 99% for those diagnosed with cancer limited to the breast. Even for those patients with lymph node involvement, five-year survival is 86% (77% among black women). These numbers obviously point to racial disparity, a troubling issue under intensive investigation. Although only about 4–6% of newly diagnosed patients have metastatic disease (MBC), their five-year survival was 27% (20% among black women). These patients are sometimes referred to as having de novo metastatic breast cancer (2).

As a dramatic sign of progress, it should be noted that the overall mortality from breast cancer has decreased by 40% since 1989 (2).

Much research has been devoted to trying to understand the racial disparities listed above, including socioeconomic issues, insurance status, access to healthcare, comorbidities, diet, and innumerable other factors. However, it appears that one of the major disparities is in tumor biology, with more black women developing aggressive variants of breast cancer such as triple-negative disease (5, 6)

When one thinks of the number of patients just in the United States at risk for the development of MBC, we should realize that currently there are over 3,861,500 breast cancer survivors (7), virtually any of whom could ultimately develop MBC. Fortunately, while a large percentage of these women have likely been cured, relapses (especially among the 70% of women whose tumors were estrogen-receptor positive) can occur late, even at ten, fifteen, twenty, or even more years after their original diagnosis. It has been estimated that 150,000 breast cancer survivors are living with MBC, three-quarters of whom were originally diagnosed with stage I to III breast cancers (7). The following table breaks down the almost 4 million survivors by age of diagnosis and years since diagnosis (6).

Age at Diagnosis (%)	Year Since Diagnosis (%)
<50 (7)	<5 (29)
50 to 64 (29)	5 to 10 (23)
65 to 84 (51)	10 to 15 (17)
85+ (13)	15 to 20 (12)
	>20 (19)

While survival statistics have steadily increased over the decades for MBC, they have been less dramatic than for early-stage disease and the cure barrier has not yet been breached.

In 1992, our group published a series of 193 patients treated at the University of Miami (FL) between 1986 and 1992 and reviewed the world's literature of similar series prior to 1992. The median survival from first relapse (MSFR) was twenty-six months, not dissimilar to nineteen other published series from the 1980s to early 1990s (8).

In 2015, Zeichner, publishing for our group, studied the MSFR for 189 patients treated between 1996 and 2006, with the result being thirty-three months (seven months better than our previous study two decades earlier). Likewise, our literature review revealed nine additional publications over this time frame again with largely similar results to our own (9).

In our literature review, the paper by Giordano at MD Anderson Cancer stood out as a major outlier (10) with a MSFR of fifty-eight months. This series of 106 patients included patients with local-regional relapse, a group known to have a more favorable prognosis than patients with metastases to bone, liver, lung, etc. Such patients were excluded from our publication because a finite percentage of those patients can actually be cured. The reader is directed to chapter 3 of this book where we highlight five such patients, likely cured of their local-regional cancer recurrence in the breast or nearby lymph nodes.

Zeichner went one step further and separately analyzed 153 patients with de novo MBC (distant metastases diagnosed at the same time their primary breast cancer was discovered) (11). As previously mentioned, these patients constitute only 4–6% of all patients with MBC. This analysis included two different groups of patients, one from the University of Miami and one from the same breast-cancer specific private practice analyzed in the last paragraph. Regardless, the results were quite similar to the larger group of patients with MBC. Although the end points used in the two Zeichner trials were slightly different (median survival from first relapse) MSFR for MBC without de novo MBC and overall survival for the de novo series, the MSFR of thirty-three months is not dissimilar to the thirty-six months overall survival for the University of Miami de novo series or the forty-one months overall survival for the private practice series.

In summary, with regard to survival statistics, we know that survival for MBC patients was less than 2 years prior to 1990, two years or better in the 1990s and early 2000s and closer to three years by about 2006. As of 2020 (statistics available through about 2015), the authors would not be surprised if the overall survival in newer series approaches four to five years.

Improvements in outcomes have been accomplished while also diminishing the toxic impact of the therapies themselves. The radical mastectomy (radical removal of the breast) performed in the 1960s and earlier is largely a procedure of the past, and it has repeatedly been proven that simple removal of the breast lump (tumor) followed by radiation of the breast is at least equivalent to breast removal in terms of ultimate outcomes when lumpectomy is an option. Even if breast removal is required, advances in breast reconstruction techniques over time have led to less deformity.

Complete axillary dissection (removal of the lymph nodes in the armpit/axilla) was also a standard surgical procedure in the 1960s and 1970s and is associated with a 30% risk of swelling of the arm (lymphedema). See Beth's story (chapter 7). Today, the use of sentinel node biopsy has markedly reduced the use of axillary dissection, thus further reducing the morbidity of breast cancer surgery.

While many patients require radiation therapy after lumpectomy (or sometimes even after mastectomy), technology has become far more sophisticated and safer over the last several decades. Additionally, the number of radiation treatments needed has been reduced from five to six weeks of daily dosing (M–F) to three to four weeks, and in some cases, radiation may be delivered over one to five treatments.

Although chemotherapy (strong drugs) is commonly used before or after surgery for early-stage breast cancer, advances in genetic prognostic tests such as Oncotype DX, MammaPrint, and others have reduced the use of chemotherapy in early-stage breast cancer by about 20% (12). However, chemotherapy (of many different types) remains an important tool in our armamentarium against MBC.

The doctors primarily charged with treating MBC are called medical oncologists. However, MBC may require the expertise of surgical and/or radiation oncologists as part of the multidisciplinary team. While early-stage breast cancer almost always requires this multidisciplinary team, there are many situations in MBC that benefit from surgical and radiation oncology expertise as well.

In general, the medical oncologist is the captain of the ship for patients with MBC and is responsible for making decisions regarding classical chemotherapy drugs, antihormonal agents, and when available, targeted agents to control this disease. As of 2021, immunotherapy approaches have also been approved for select situations within MBC. Treatment strategies, whenever possible, should utilize least toxic drugs available and emphasize quality of life. Fortunately, 70% of patients have tumors that are estrogen-receptor positive and HER2 negative (see definitions on next page). The majority of these patients can be managed, at least initially, with relatively nontoxic antihormone pills. This may be combined with one of the novel targeted CDK4/6 inhibitors, which are also administered by mouth. Thus, the majority of MBC patients can often be managed initially with minimally toxic oral agents.

Who *needs* chemotherapy as initial therapy for MBC:

1. Estrogen-receptor-positive patients with rapidly progressive disease such as involvement of liver or lungs, or widespread bone metastases, which cause significant and unrelenting pain. Fortunately, these situations are relatively uncommon in patients with MBC.
2. Triple-negative MBC.
3. HER2 positive MBC (in combination with anti-HER2 targeted agents).

At this point, the above paragraph got a little ahead of itself using technical terms that have not yet been described to the reader. For that reason, the following sections will provide the definitions of some of the medical terms used throughout this book.

Biomarkers: Substances that doctors test for in all breast cancer patients and help to define the potential prognosis of a patient's particular cancer and provide information as to how best to treat the disease. The three most important biomarkers are estrogen receptor (ER), progesterone receptor (PR), and HER2/neu (H-2-N). These three biomarkers along with other highly sophisticated tests, which include large numbers of genes, allowed scientists to describe four major subtypes of breast cancer (13, 14). Additional subtypes are being discovered, and in time, we will likely discover how unique every breast cancer is in each individual patient. For now, however, for simplicity we shall define the following:

1. Luminal A: (ER and/or PR positive and H-2-N negative). These tumors tend to have the best prognosis.
2. Luminal B: Same biomarkers as luminal A, but with a much less favorable prognosis.
3. HER2/neu positive: These tumors may be either ER and/or PR positive or ER and/or PR negative but contain too many copies of the HER2 gene. Patients whose tumors contain ER, PR, and HER2/neu are often referred to as triple positive. Since the discovery of drugs targeting HER2 (e.g., Herceptin and others), triple-positive patients are emerging as a specific subgroup with a good prognosis. ER and PR negative and HER2/neu positive patients also have a far better prognosis than in the past.
4. Triple-negative (TNBC): These tumors are negative for ER, PR, and HER2/neu. The other three subtypes have specific drugs

which target the biomarkers in question, e.g., antihormones for ER/PR positive (luminal A and B tumors) or trastuzumab (Herceptin), lapatinib (Tykerb), ado-trastuzumab emtansine (Kadcyla) neratinib, tucatinib, and Enhertu for HER2-positive disease. Unfortunately, no such reproducible target currently exists for triple-negative disease. Hence, for the moment, chemotherapy is the only option for triple-negative MBC, and it has the least favorable prognosis of all the subtypes. Immunotherapy is looking promising for some patients with TNBC.

TNBC is a heterogeneous population. Researchers at Vanderbilt University (15, 16) and others have subdivided TNBC into four or more subtypes with different degrees of biologic behavior from aggressive to indolent. Within the next few years, TNBC is likely to be further subdivided as we learn more about the mutations driving each subtype. Therefore, new targeted therapies can be developed to attack the mutation driving the multiplication of tumor cells in that particular cancer.

Many patients with TNBC have been found to be carriers of specific genetic mutations called BRCA 1 and 2. While BRCA carriers will often have TNBC, BRCA carriers may also have luminal or even HER2-positive breast cancer. Fortunately, patients with BRCA mutations have a particular genetic defect that can be exploited therapeutically. These patients have a defect in PARP, a substance important in the repair of DNA. Scientists have developed PARP inhibitors, and we are using these drugs while learning how we can use them to treat BRCA carriers with MBC successfully. Ongoing clinical trials aim to determine if the use of these inhibitors in patients with early-stage breast cancer can actually cure BRCA positive cancers, when used in combination with or sequenced with other drugs. Patients with TNBC who are BRCA carriers may well respond to treatment with a PARP inhibitor. PARP inhibitors have also been shown to produce responses in BRCA-positive patients with MBC whose tumors are estrogen-receptor positive.

As each patient's clinical history contains many scientific and medical terms, it would be beyond the scope of this introduction to define them all. However, aside from the four major subtypes listed above, each chapter typically identifies the type of that person's cancer as it appears to the pathologist, the physician who studies the tumors with a microscope.

Regardless of subtype, you may see the terms *infiltrating ductal* or *infiltrating lobular carcinoma.*

Infiltrating or invasive signifies that this tumor is invading normal structures around it (hence, cancer). The breast is composed of lobules that make milk, which is carried to the nipple through ducts (tubes). Approximately 80% of breast cancers arise in the ducts (hence, infiltrating ductal), and 9 to 10% are lobular, hence infiltrating lobular. The remaining 10% of breast cancers are rare subtypes (tubular, medullary, micropapillary, mucinous, metaplastic, and many others).

Some of the patients in this book have a genetic predisposition to the development of cancer (i.e., BRCA and other genes as described above). A common misconception is that if someone has no relative with cancer that they have no risk of developing breast cancer. In fact, more than 80% of breast cancer patients have no family history, and only about 10% of patients are found to have a known gene mutation predisposing them to the disease. Before 2015, the only mutations we could test for were BRCA 1 and 2. After 2015, we began to learn about many more genes that also predispose to breast cancer. Interestingly, only half of the 10% of cancers associated with genetic mutations are BRCA1 or BRCA2 related. For that reason, many companies offer genetic panel testing encompassing from 20 to over 84 genes. We are only now beginning to learn more about the relationship of PALB2, CHEK2, PTEN, ATM, the Lynch syndrome family of genes, and others, and how they relate to breast cancer. At the present time, there are stringent guidelines utilized by insurance companies to determine who should undergo genetic testing. Unfortunately, it has been determined recently that in some large data sets, only 50% of patients found to have a deleterious mutation in a gene actually met the current guidelines for reimbursement. Thus, if the other 50% had not been tested for some reason (perhaps even financial) their genetic predisposition would not have been discovered.

Another fact about these deleterious genes, which predispose to breast cancer, is that they may also be associated with other cancers. BRCA 1 and 2 may also predispose to ovarian, pancreatic and prostate cancers as well as malignant melanoma. BRCA2 may predispose to male breast cancer. Lynch syndrome can predispose to colon or uterine cancers as well as breast cancer. Patients who are carriers of one of these mutations would be best served by counseling not only by their oncologist but also with a trained and licensed genetic counselor.

The Chapters

Each chapter in this book represents a person or multiple people who lived (or is living) far longer than the average survival for MBC or who presents an uplifting/inspiring message for the reader.

The chapters each begin with the chronology of that individual's medical history. In each case, it may prove technical for the average reader. The authors do not expect the reader to read every word of every chronology. However, the detailed information is provided for those who find your own story to be similar to a story discussed in a chapter.

If there is one takeaway message from many of these chronologies, an analogy may be found in the "The Frog Prince" fairy tale: "You've got to kiss a lot of frogs." This is true in MBC as well. When things are going poorly and the last two or three treatments have not been successful, don't despair, the next frog (treatment) could be your prince (remission).

Following each medical history, the authors will try to capture the key takeaway which may have helped each of these patients achieve a better-than-expected outcome. Lest you think the authors are taking credit for these outcomes, we are not. Many of the same treatment decisions in others have not worked as dramatically. The real answers are more evasive.

Was there something in his person's genetic makeup that led to them responding better to the same treatment provided to others? Was there something in this person's psychosocial adaptation or family support system contributing to the better outcome? What about faith and spiritual influences? See chapter 11 (Rebecca); what about true grit—that innate desire to overcome and fight and not passively accepting what appears to be a bad set of cards dealt to you? (See chapter 2, "Joan").

Hopefully, the reader will review the takeaway messages after each patient's history in which we shall endeavor to explain in layman's terms and not doctorese.

Finally, each chapter will provide the person (or family) an opportunity to discuss their own personal journey with MBC, which, we hope, will yield inspiration to those fighting or about to fight that battle.

CHAPTER II

Inspirational Stories of Patients— Not Necessarily Metastatic Breast Cancer (MBC)

Two of the three patients in this chapter do not fit the majority population portrayed in this book, which is MBC. Joan's story is that of true grit, pushing ahead with her life in spite of the stressful treatments she underwent.

Henrietta's story is a reminder that as bad as the statistics look for patients with 20 or more positive lymph nodes at primary diagnosis, long life without relapse is possible.

Kaye did have metastatic cancer and has apparently been cured even though we are not sure where her metastatic disease originated. It may have started in her breast, but it could also have been primary peritoneal cancer.

1: Joan
True Grit

Although this book is about metastatic breast cancer, it is also meant to be inspirational. While Joan was not diagnosed with metastatic breast cancer, we feel the reader will find her story inspirational.

History

Joan was a forty-one-year-old premenopausal teacher and mother. She is a dedicated and accomplished marathon runner.

Beginning in 2015, a small nodule in the left breast was followed regularly with imaging studies. However, it enlarged over time, leading to a left breast biopsy in 2018, which revealed extensive ductal carcinoma in situ (DCIS) with a 4 mm area of invasive ductal cancer that was estrogen receptor 92% positive, progesterone receptor 30% positive, HER-2 negative, and with a high Ki-67 (test of aggressiveness of the tumor). MRI measurement was 6.6 cm by 5.8 cm.

Two different opinions were rendered. The first was for chemotherapy prior to surgery, and the second was for bilateral mastectomies. The patient was not comfortable with either recommendation initially and sought another opinion with us. As the tumor was estrogen-receptor positive, during our first visit, she accepted the concept of trying to shrink the tumor with antihormonal therapy (tamoxifen).

Unfortunately, after a month of tamoxifen, the tumor actually increased in size. By that time, she had acclimatized to the prospect of bilateral mastectomies with reconstruction as her best option.

Upon review of the pathology, while the right breast was completely negative, there was 4.5 cm area of DCIS (90% of the tumor) and twenty separate areas of microscopic invasion. Additionally, the sentinel node was positive for cancer on the left side, leading to removal of seventeen more lymph nodes, all of which were negative. The tumor was found to be MammaPrint luminal B, indicating that postoperative chemotherapy could be beneficial.

Joan was recommended Taxotere and Cytoxan chemotherapy for four doses (one every three weeks) to be followed by postmastectomy radiation and then antihormonal therapy.

She experienced complications including infection of her expander implant reconstruction. Ultimately, she achieved an excellent cosmetic result prior to starting chemotherapy. While our office was geographically far from her home, we had the availability of a scalp cooling device to attempt hair preservation during chemotherapy. She decided to proceed with chemotherapy at our institution and was able to preserve her hair.

On her last day of treatment, Joan said, "You know, this chemo wasn't so bad. There is a 50K run tomorrow, and I'm going to run." And run she did, coming in as the first woman runner to finish the 50K.

Radiation therapy was next, and after finishing radiation, she said, "Radiation wasn't so bad. There's a 100K this weekend and I'm going to run". And run she did, coming in first among the leaders.

Postscript

After radiation, Joan stared on Zoladex, a drug to ensure that she would be postmenopausal, and started the antihormone, letrozole.

Finally, she elected to participate in a clinical trial aimed at finding out whether aspirin would contribute to the curability of early-stage breast cancer. She elected to be randomized to an aspirin 325 mg/day or 81 mg/day or a placebo. Joan, being Joan, wanted to contribute by participating in a clinical trial to find the answer to the aspirin question which could help the next generation of women fighting breast cancer.

1, Joan: Takeaway

Joan epitomizes the strength and resilience of women faced with a serious but curable medical condition. The cure rate of early-stage breast cancer like Joan's is high but achieved with the use of multiple treatments each of which may have unpleasant side effects.

Joan had both breasts removed and experienced severe infections during reconstruction. However, she and her surgeons persevered, and she has an excellent cosmetic outcome.

As for chemotherapy, her use of scalp cooling resulted in no significant hair loss. Twelve weeks of chemotherapy did not interfere significantly with her quality of life, and she placed first in a 50K marathon the day after her fourth dose of chemotherapy. Likewise, radiation therapy was just another inconvenience between her 50K and 100K marathon successes.

Her therapy put her into menopause through chemotherapy and then chemical suppression of her ovaries, followed by initiation of at least five years of the aromatase inhibitor antihormone letrozole. While natural menopause or artificially induced early menopause can be associated with quality-of-life changes, we are sure that Joan will handle these changes with the same glowing smile and natural radiance that she exhibited throughout the earlier and tougher segments of her therapeutic journey.

Outrunning Cancer: Joan's Story

It was a beautiful Florida evening, and I was finishing up a sunset run on some local trails. I was focused on the deep breaths, decompressing from my day of teaching elementary school, and full of thankfulness for this time to get out and get exercise. My four kids were home working on homework, and I relished a few minutes by myself in nature.

The phone rang, breaking the stillness of the woods.

On the other end of the line was my oncologist, Dr. Vogel. Over the last months, his impact on my life had become extraordinary in so many ways, and I answered with a very cheery, "Hey, Doc! What's up?"

He proceeded to tell me how amazed he was to learn I had completed a 50K (32 mile) race a few days earlier. Running a long-distance race wasn't new to me, but the fact that I completed it *the day after* my last chemotherapy treatment seemed extraordinary to him.

Extraordinary. This is how I will describe my life after being diagnosed with cancer. It has been a time of perseverance, staying positive, and surrounding myself with the people who support me. It has been a time of outrunning cancer.

Perseverance. I have been an athlete most of my life. In adulthood, I became recreationally competitive as a distance runner, completing almost thirty marathons and a few 50K races. I have traveled to the big races in Chicago, New York, and Boston. My times were excellent and often resulted in wins at local and regional races. I felt in control of my body and my health and learned to persevere in order to cross finish line.

Nothing tested this perseverance like the diagnosis of breast cancer, which brought the unforeseen path of frequent doctor visits, surgical procedures, chemotherapy, radiation, and ongoing drug therapy. There were times it would have been understandable to say, "Enough is enough!" But I never did. When I felt like crawling, I walked. When I wanted to walk, I ran. It takes a great deal of determination to stay strong and put forth the effort to get through the treatments. Perseverance is key.

I knew I had to keep my thoughts and goals in a positive, upbeat mode! Cancer can certainly take from you—days you don't feel well, the time it takes to go to appointments, and missing out on life events because you're recovering from treatments. I promised myself that I would not allow the negative parts of cancer to consume one more minute of my time than necessary. With every step, I kept (and continue to keep) a positive mindset! I am strong! I'm doing everything I can to stay healthy! Others were watching. It was time to be an extraordinary example of showing joy in the journey.

Yes, there were times when the tears flowed. I was tired of being sidelined when I wanted to be on adventures with my kids or back at my classroom. My running friends headed to the Boston Marathon while I recovered from a surgery, and I fantasized about sneaking away and doing the race anyway. Reminding myself to stay positive was essential. This was all a temporary setback, and I was going to get back to everything soon enough! I would take this life speed bump a day at a time with a positive heart.

No one wants cancer. However, if I had to go through it, I didn't want to waste it. This would be a time to grow my faith in God and to discover my strength. I would invest in relationships with other pink sisters and be an inspiration to those around me. A whole community, including my children, were watching me on this journey as I outran cancer.

Two years later, I can tell you that I have not only reclaimed my life, but it has been restored to more than I imagined. I'm active in every part of my kids' lives, my students still call me their favorite teacher, I took up a hobby of backpacking in the mountains, and yes, I'm running consistently. Recent marathons include New York; Washington, DC (Marine Corps Marathon); and Boston—*twice*! I sent my oncologist a photo of the finish line of the first Boston post-treatment, texting, "This one is for you!"

Part way through chemotherapy treatments, I decided I needed a big dream and goal to help me persevere and stay positive. I signed up for a 100-mile race called Ancient Oaks, which is held in December in Northern Florida. I kept that race in mind as I faced the difficult days. It got me out the door and training when others might have said I had the right to stay at home and "take care of myself."

After my last session of radiation was complete, I ran the 100-mile race and *won* it! It took me about twenty-five hours, but I was smiling most of the time. Other runners knew my story, and they encouraged me as much as I inspired them. The finish line was crowded with close friends and family. One hundred miles! More than I could have imagined. It has been an extraordinary journey. I took my chance to persevere and stay positive, and to outrun cancer.

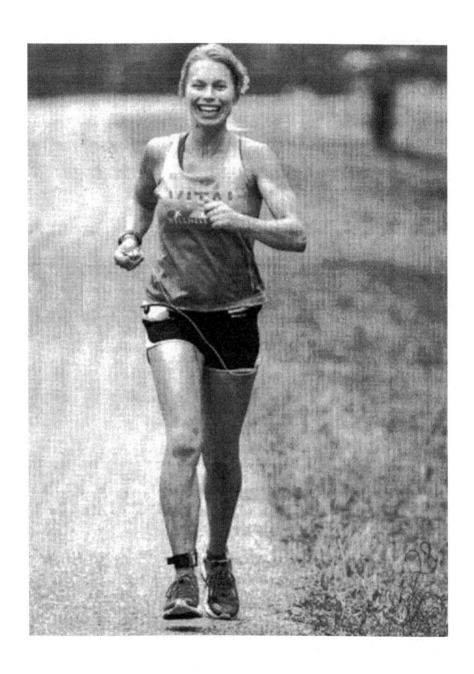

2: Henrietta

At age fifty-six in 1987, Henrietta underwent a right lumpectomy for breast cancer and was found to have twenty-four involved lymph nodes. Luckily, she had no distant spread of cancer. Though her treatment records are no longer available, we know that she received an aggressive form of Adriamycin-based chemotherapy. Incidentally, her surgeon, who was a world-renowned oncologic surgeon, did not want her to undergo radiation therapy. In the current era, this would be a major deviation from standard of care. She would have been recommended radiation to both the breast and the regional lymph nodes.

Genetic testing performed years later when the technology became available was negative. However, she did have a variant of uncertain significance in one gene known as the ATM gene. As variants of uncertain significance do not have any clinical relevance currently, her results would not lead to any intervention either for Henrietta or her family members.

She received eleven years of tamoxifen after chemotherapy without radiation therapy and is now *thirty-five years disease-free.*

2, Henrietta: Takeaway

At least twenty to thirty times each year, I encounter patients with very large tumors or a large number of involved lymph nodes. Invariably, the patient will ask, "Do you have any patients like me who have survived?" Henrietta is just one of many such patients who are cured of their disease. This is a result of advances in chemotherapy and hormonal therapy. Although this book is devoted to patients with MBC, I felt that those patients with advanced-stage breast cancer at diagnosis who would typically have a dire prognosis should be represented as a result of the dramatic improvement in their prognosis over the years.

3: Kaye

In 1984, at age thirty-nine, Kaye presented with an unusual clinical picture. She was diagnosed with twenty-two axillary lymph nodes involved with cancer, including supraclavicular lymph nodes. However, no tumor was discovered in her breast. Of note, the lymph nodes were found to contain psammoma bodies. She also had cancer in the abdomen and an elevated CA-125, a marker usually associated with ovarian cancer. It was unclear as to the diagnosis. Did she have an occult breast cancer that spread to the abdomen, an occult ovarian primary, or a primary peritoneal carcinoma metastatic to the lymph nodes under her arm (axillary) and above her collarbone (supraclavicular)?

She underwent extensive surgical procedures after completing aggressive preoperative treatment targeting both ovarian and breast cancer.

Kaye received a combination of Cytoxan, Adriamycin, and cisplatin followed by methotrexate and 5-FU. Subsequently, she underwent left breast and lymph node radiation, as well as a supraclavicular lymph node dissection. This was not a typical procedure at that time and would remain an unusual aspect of surgical care even today.

When she was originally diagnosed in 1984, genetic testing was not available. However, over time, she was treated for malignant melanoma of the right forearm and at that time underwent genetic testing. She was found to be a BRCA1 carrier. Her daughter is also a carrier, and Kaye's mother has subsequently developed breast cancer.

Kaye remains alive and well as of June 2020, thirty-six years after her diagnosis of metastatic cancer from an unknown primary site. This was possibly an occult breast, an ovarian primary or even primary peritoneal carcinoma in a BRCA1 carrier.

3, Kaye: Takeaway

At the time of diagnosis, Kaye was an enigma. Her disease was found in fluid within her abdomen and in lymph nodes under her arm and above her collarbone. The presence of psammoma bodies within her tumor is usually associated with ovarian carcinoma rather than breast cancer. Regardless, thirty-six years ago, she was treated aggressively for both breast and ovarian cancer. She was noted to have intra-abdominal tumor cells, and thus her cancer is best characterized as metastatic disease at diagnosis.

As no tumor was found in the breast, she did not undergo breast surgery. She did have her uterus and ovaries removed, but no cancer was identified. In case there was an occult tumor in her breast, she did receive radiation to the breast. Additionally, she received radiation to lymph nodes above the collarbone and in the axilla.

The diagnosis of melanoma later in life further hinted that she could be a BRCA carrier, as that gene can predict for breast, ovarian, prostate, and pancreatic tumors, as well as melanoma. Indeed, she did test positive for the BRCA1 gene, which then led to the discovery of the gene in her daughter. This discovery provided the knowledge that she could develop cancer in the future, and it allowed her to take appropriate preventative actions.

Kaye's Story

I am so happy and honored to share my success story.

A new chapter of my life began on July 11, 1982, when I remarried and moved from NYC to Miami Beach with my nine-year-old daughter, Amanda. Dan and I had just celebrated our marriage with a wonderful wedding at the United Nations Plaza Hotel, and we were excited to start our new life together in Florida.

Dan's two children, Lori (twenty-three and working in Miami) and Doug (twenty and studying hard at UF), were most welcoming to Amanda and me. We settled into Dan's apartment but soon realized that we needed more space. We bought a home with a pool on a golf course in Hollywood, Florida. What New Yorker wouldn't love that? We had room to spread out and begin making new memories. The days of barbeques and pool parties were awesome. I had been a teacher in New York at a private boy's school, a job I loved. However, in Florida, Dan had his own mortgage company. I wanted to work alongside him, so I obtained my mortgage license, and we joined forces. It was during those very happy honeymoon days that I first noticed a lump on the side of my neck.

Checking it out, we were first told that it was most likely an infection from recent dental work. *Not so!* That was the beginning of my Orwellian nightmare.

Subsequent biopsies showed papillary cells with psammoma bodies. Perhaps I had thyroid cancer? Almost overnight, a large mass of lymph nodes formed under my left arm. A biopsy revealed metastatic cells from either breast, lung, or ovaries, but *no* tumor—*no* primary. Still searching for answers, I had an oophorectomy (removal of my ovaries) with abdominal washing three times. Pathology again showed metastatic disease, but no primary site.

Without a primary being found, it was suggested that I begin a regimen of chemo—the big guns! I began doing my own research regarding diet, nutritional supplementation, and meditation. I wanted to combine that with my chemo protocol. It was a very scary time. My mother had died from breast cancer at fifty-six. I watched as the chemo debilitated her, and I did not want to be that person. I resolved to do *anything* and *everything* in my power to stay alive.

After three months of very heavy chemo, I passed out in my house and required two pints of blood. Chemotherapy was stopped, and I underwent six weeks of radiation concomitant with oral chemo. My body was depleted, but I stayed the course.

I continued my path of wellness toward recovery using all the resources from my doctors, my friends, and my family. It was a very rough and uncertain two-year journey. I continued with regular checkups, lab studies evaluating tumor markers, and praying. Somehow, I continued to get better and stronger.

Today, thirty-six years later, we are a loving family. All three children are married and have enriched our lives with seven amazing grandchildren, ages sixteen to thirty-four. I could have missed all of that! We have been on trips and cruises together celebrating life's milestones. My life has truly been blessed.

About fifteen years ago, we sold the empty-nest house and moved into a high-rise condominium in downtown Fort Lauderdale. We can walk to restaurants, museums, retail shops, art galleries, and the performing arts theater. It's so alive and vibrant. We can watch the warm healing sun rise each morning over the Atlantic Ocean, then settle into its resting place each evening with a magnificent colorful display over the Everglades.

It is my tiny little slice of NYC; I have come full circle.

I owe my happiness to my family, especially my husband, the love of my life. I could not have made it without him!

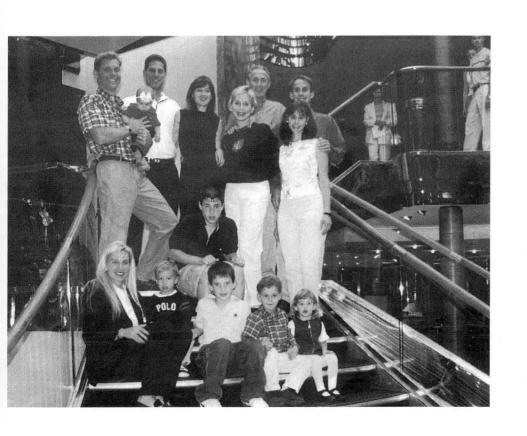

CHAPTER III

Stage IV NED (No Evidence of Disease) And Local Regional Recurrence

Introduction

Stage IV NED and Local regional recurrence (LRR) is a somewhat different concept from MBC. These classifications include patients who have a single or perhaps two metastatic sites that could be within the breast or chest wall after surgical resection of tumor or the breast. Additionally, the site of disease could be within regional lymph nodes, which include axillary (armpit), supraclavicular (above the collarbone), or internal mammary (inside the chest adjacent to the breastbone). When extending the definition to include single lesions in bone, brain, liver, or lung, this situation is called oligometastatic. Stage IV NED includes patients whose site of disease spread is either resected or treated with resolution if the abnormality.

Unfortunately, although there have been several attempts to mount controlled, randomized trials to determine if chemotherapy is beneficial in all cases of management of LRR, to date, only one has successfully completed patient accrual. That study (17), CALOR, randomized patients after local regional treatment for a local or regional recurrence to chemotherapy or no chemotherapy. Patients with estrogen-receptor-positive disease also received antihormonal therapy. The results indicated a statistically significant 10% benefit to chemotherapy for estrogen-receptor-negative patients but results in estrogen-receptor positive (most of whom also received hormonal therapy) were not significant. While providing some hints as to treatment strategies, the number of patients in this trial were far smaller than the typical trials we usually rely upon to make definitive treatment decisions.

The MD Anderson group has published sequential, nonrandomized trials (18) in these patients. They routinely take an aggressive approach and treat with curative intent in this patient population. This included patients with isolated visceral (organ based) metastasis. However, in the absence of appropriate controlled randomized trials, the effectiveness of these aggressive strategies remains uncertain.

Regardless, it is likely that a large percentage of patients with local regional relapse have a better prognosis than classical MBC patients who have recurrence outside of the local regional area (19) when treated appropriately.

1: Amy

Amy underwent bilateral mastectomies with reconstruction in 2002 at age forty-six for ductal carcinoma in situ of the left breast. The right mastectomy was prophylactic. No further treatment was given.

In June 2006, she developed a mass under the left arm and had removal of the left axillary node showing metastatic cancer. This was followed by an axillary dissection (removal of all the lymph nodes under the arm) and removal of the chest muscle. The remainder of the lymph nodes were negative, and a metastatic workup, which looks for disease elsewhere in the body, was negative. The positive lymph node was ER and PR negative and HER2/neu positive.

The patient was treated in the local recurrence setting with Adriamycin followed by Taxol and Herceptin and then local-regional radiation, which involved radiation to the chest wall and regional lymph nodes. Herceptin, a drug to treat HER2/neu positive disease was continued for a full year and completed on August 30, 2007.

Amy is disease-free as of 2020, fourteen years after her recurrence.

Amy's takeaway points will appear later in this chapter.

Amy's Story

Being diagnosed in 2002 (with DCIS) was very scary. I was a single mom of thirteen- and ten-year-old sons. I worked full time as a prekindergarten teacher. I followed my doctor's plan and had a bilateral mastectomy with reconstruction. It was determined at the time that no other course of action was necessary. The thought that I was cancer-free was very good.

In 2006, a recurrence in chest wall and lymph nodes was discovered on the same side as the original cancer. It was a shock to me, not only to my body, but to my entire being. I can remember thinking, "Oh no, I had better get my affairs in order," just like I'd seen in so many movies with a cancer diagnosis in their story lines. What followed was meeting Dr. Vogel and a very aggressive treatment approach that included surgery, fifty-two weeks of chemo, and eight weeks of radiation. What also followed were many questions, such as "Will I be here to see my boys graduate from high school and college?" "Will I be at their weddings?" "Will I live to enjoy my grandchildren?" I had some very dark thoughts and feelings during this time. I had always been known among friends and family for my positive attitude and high energy level (I'm an avid walker and spent most weekends enjoying a local 5K). I did my very best to continue to be me, despite significant nausea, fatigue, sadness, and worry.

Dr. Vogel and his staff were highly professional, kind, and compassionate. My family was so supportive. My parents took me to every single chemo treatment, and I'm forever thankful. My friends and colleagues at school were helpful and cheerful, and kept me laughing and sane. I'll always remember their care and concern. My boys and I went through this together. Besides cancer, I was going through a tough divorce. I was fighting a few battles. I wanted to show my boys that when life knocks you on your butt, you get up, brush yourself off, and keep moving forward!

Since reading Dr. Vogel's book, I've been thinking so much about him and my time in his care. With every patient Dr. Vogel treats, he touches so many lives—all his patients, their families, their friends, and their support systems. By now, due to his fantastic career, he's touched the lives of many thousands of people.

In my career as a teacher, I hope that my legacy is far reaching as well. I teach prekindergarten; I teach reading, writing, math, science, and social studies. More importantly, I teach kindness, patience, love, respect, and acceptance. These are the life lessons that I hope will follow my students when they leave my class, the gifts that I hope make a difference in their lives. I teach them to love themselves and to take that love and spread it all around! Cancer changed me in so many ways—as a woman, a mother, and a teacher. I've spent more time thinking about what matters most in my life, and I am so very grateful for the time I was given time to see my boys grow to be amazing men, time to touch more lives in the classroom, and time to enjoy the little things, such as reading, walking outdoors in nature, and being a student of life.

I am almost sixty-five years old; I've been teaching for close to thirty years. I have been cancer free for fourteen years. My sons are now thirty-two and twenty-nine years old. Both have successful careers. My older son is married to the love of his life, and they have a three-year-old son, whom I adore; he calls me "Nana!" My younger son is getting married in a couple of months, and I'm looking forward to another wonderful celebration. I'm still an avid walker; I walk every day, sometimes twice a day, and on occasion, three times a day! I've been thankful for Dr. Vogel every day since I met him. I'm thankful for the gift that is my life.

"I don't want my life to be defined by what is etched on my tombstone. I want it to be defined in what is etched in the lives and hearts of those I've touched" (Steve Maraboli).

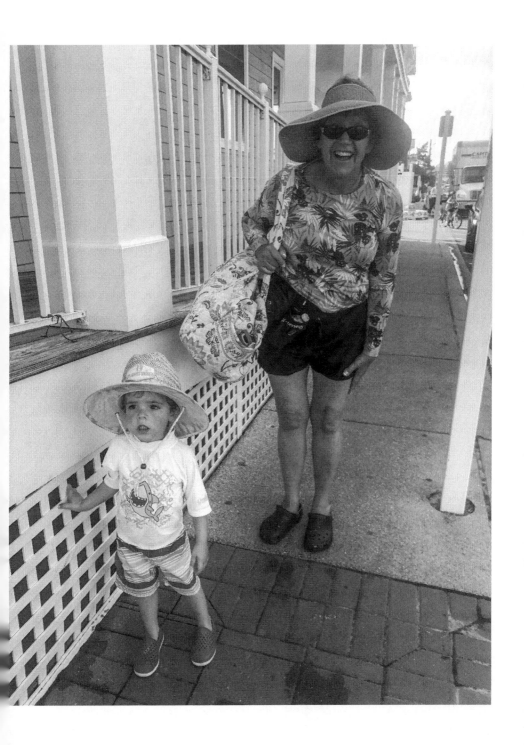

2: Fathemeh

In the year 2000, at age forty, Fathemeh was diagnosed with right-sided ductal carcinoma in situ treated with lumpectomy, radiation, tamoxifen, and then anastrozole.

She was found to be BRCA2 positive and underwent removal of her uterus, fallopian tubes, and ovaries.

At age forty-seven, Fathemeh developed locally recurrent invasive right breast cancer. She underwent bilateral mastectomies with the left being prophylactic. Her final pathology showed high-grade ductal carcinoma in situ with no evidence of residual invasive disease. This indicated that the diagnostic core biopsy removed all her primary invasive cancer. However, she was noted to have two of twenty-two lymph nodes involved with cancer. Her tumor was triple negative. This means that it is ER and PR negative, as well as HER2 negative. Adjuvant chemotherapy consisting of dose dense Adriamycin and Cytoxan was followed by Taxol. The term *dose dense* means that the Adriamycin and Cytoxan is given every two weeks instead of every three weeks, which is the typical schedule. Dose dense treatment was accomplished with the use of the drug pegfilgrastim (Neulasta) to bring the white blood count up quickly to allow therapy every two weeks. Radiation was not recommended as she had previously received it in 2000.

Fathemeh remains disease-free as of the year 2020, thirteen years after the diagnosis of recurrence.

1 and 2, Amy and Fathemeh: Takeaway

These two patients have one major similarity but other significant differences. Both had an invasive breast cancer local or regional recurrence *after* an initial diagnosis of DCIS. As noted in the introduction, recurrences after DCIS are relatively rare, and death after an initial diagnosis of DCIS occurs in only 3% of patients with a diagnosis of DCIS. However, we know that 50% of recurrences after DCIS are not DCIS but are invasive cancers. Amy and Fatemeh are two such patients who experienced invasive recurrences. Fortunately, both are cancer free thirteen and fourteen years after their recurrences, respectively.

Initial diagnosis of DCIS was the only common thread between these two patients as Amy developed an estrogen-receptor negative and HER2 positive recurrence, and Fathemeh had a triple-negative recurrence and was a BRCA2 carrier. Both women received Adriamycin and Cytoxan chemotherapy followed by Taxol, with Herceptin appropriately added to Amy's regimen.

Given that the great majority of late relapses (beyond ten years) occur in ER positive tumors and both of these women's invasive tumors were ER negative, I believe that we can be optimistic that they are likely to be cured of their recurrent cancers.

3: Patricia

At age sixty-one, in June 2002, Patricia developed an ER negative and PR negative inflammatory breast cancer that was HER2 positive. She was treated with chemotherapy initially (neoadjuvant), receiving carboplatin, Taxol, and sixteen doses of Herceptin. This was followed by four cycles of FEC (five fluorouracil-epirubicin and cytoxan). She subsequently underwent a left mastectomy. Microscopic residual disease was found in three of eleven lymph nodes, and she then received nineteen additional Herceptin doses to complete one full year.

Comprehensive radiation therapy was delivered in 2003 while undergoing Herceptin therapy.

In January 2004, eight months after completion of Herceptin therapy, a left chest wall recurrence developed. She did not receive any additional surgery, radiation, or chemotherapy. Herceptin alone was recommended and has been continued since that time (sixteen years), with no further evidence of recurrent disease.

On several occasions, we have raised the question of whether or not Patricia would consider the possibility of stopping the Herceptin, yet each time, she has declined.

3, Patricia: Takeaway

Patricia constitutes an ongoing dilemma for herself, and other patients like her as well as their oncologist. The reader will encounter several other women in subsequent chapters. Is it possible that some individuals with metastatic HER2 positive cancers are *cured* of their disease and is it therefore safe to stop maintenance Herceptin after some undefined, but finite period of time (21)? The answer to the dilemma remains unclear, and treatment recommendations remain individualized.

Patricia is now sixteen years since diagnosis of an inflammatory-like skin recurrence on her chest wall. She fears that stopping Herceptin will result in her cancer returning. Unfortunately, as of 2020, medical science has no answer to this question, and Patricia dutifully returns to clinic every three weeks for Herceptin treatment. Under similar circumstances, others have discontinued Herceptin and remained disease-free (see chapter 7, "Andrea"). Other women have stopped Herceptin and their cancers have recurred. Finally, some women who have had prolonged periods of disease control have decided to discontinue Herceptin while in remission. We all hope that their decision to discontinue will do as well as Andrea.

What a conundrum for doctors and patients alike.

4: Laura

At age fifty-five, Laura underwent a left mastectomy in 1988. This was for a cancer that was presumably estrogen-receptor positive with negative nodes. She received tamoxifen postoperatively.

Laura developed a chest wall recurrence on top of her expander implant in 1989, which was estrogen receptor negative. The recurrence was surgically removed, and she subsequently received Adriamycin and Cytoxan, followed by CMF chemotherapy. CMF chemotherapy was a common regimen in 1989 but is used less frequently today, although it appears to be particularly active in triple-negative breast cancer. She completed treatment with radiation.

On May 3, 2016, the badly encapsulated implant had silicone leakage and was removed. She is not desirous of further reconstruction.

It has now been thirty years since diagnosis of breast cancer with aggressive treatment of a local recurrence, and she continues to be disease-free.

4, Laura: Takeaway

Laura is an example of a patient apparently cured after diagnosis of local recurrence of breast cancer. As noted in the introduction to this chapter, patients with local or regional recurrences of breast cancer have a better prognosis than those with recurrences in some other site such as bone, liver, lung, etc. Whether these recurrences need to be treated aggressively with systemic agents such as chemotherapy in addition to local and regional modalities (surgery and radiation) still remains speculative. The literature presents a wide variation in freedom from systemic relapse with local regional therapies, ranging from a fifteen-year survival of 12% presented by MD Anderson Cancer Center in their first stage IV NED manuscript (18), to 26–69% in more recent series (19, 20).

Whether the aggressive chemotherapy regimens we gave Laura in 1989 contributed to her probable cure is unknown to this day. Surgical removal of isolated single recurrences in triple-negative breast cancers, even without systemic therapy, have resulted in long-term disease control (see chapter 9), and thus it is unclear if the chemotherapy was of benefit.

5: Anonymous

At age fifty-four, in the mid-1980s, this woman underwent a left mastectomy and then received tamoxifen for about seven years. Details of the diagnosis are unknown.

About a year after tamoxifen was discontinued, she developed a biopsy proven inflammatory recurrence in the skin overlying the reconstructed left breast. This was treated with radiation and reinstitution of tamoxifen. Tamoxifen continued for eight years and was discontinued in the early 2020's. She was then worked up for what was thought to be metastatic disease to the bone. Ultimately, it was discovered that she had an osteoporotic stress fracture. Over the years, her issues have been related to osteoporosis and not cancer.

She has received no specific antineoplastic therapy since discontinuing Tamoxifen and is recurrence-free for over twenty years after inflammatory carcinoma recurrence in her left chest wall.

5, Anonymous: Takeaway

This patient's local recurrence was an inflammatory type, which is usually associated with a poor prognosis. After biopsy, she received radiation and restarted tamoxifen. At this point, it is unclear why she did not receive chemotherapy, but our intent was to continue tamoxifen indefinitely or until relapse. However, she was taken off the drug after eight years as it was felt that she was relapsing in bone. However, as previously noted, her issue was actually severe osteoporosis. After stopping tamoxifen, she received no further anticancer therapy and has been disease free over twenty years after her inflammatory breast cancer local recurrence. Was she cured by radiation therapy? Did tamoxifen add to her salvage radiation? No one can be certain, but we are all thankful for the outcome.

CHAPTER IV

Breast Cancer with Metastases to the Ovary

(Krukenberg Tumor)

This was added as a separate chapter though ovarian metastases are not a very common entity. This decision was made as the three patients seen in recent years have all experienced encouraging clinical courses. It is noted that a series from Quebec reported on sixty-four patients treated with ovarian metastases between 1951 and 1987. In this larger series, the median survival after diagnosis of ovarian metastases was only sixteen months (22). Of course, much has changed in the treatment of MBC since the 1950s–1980s. However, the survival of Gloria (seven-plus years), Terrie (fifteen-plus years), and Barbara (twenty years) defy most MBC statistics.

1: Gloria

At age fifty-three, in December 2003, Gloria underwent a right lumpectomy for an invasive lobular carcinoma. However, because of multicentricity (spots of tumor in different quadrants of the breast), a mastectomy was performed. She did not proceed with reconstruction. The sentinel nodes were negative, and it was both estrogen receptor and HER2 positive.

Adjuvant Adriamycin and Cytoxan followed by Taxotere plus Herceptin was given, with Herceptin continuing for a year. After completion of the Taxotere, anastrozole was started but discontinued in June 2013 after 10 years of use.

Shortly after anastrozole was discontinued in 2013, Gloria was noted to have a rise in CEA (a tumor marker in the blood), and an ultrasound showed an ovarian mass. At surgery, her right ovary and fallopian tube revealed ER positive and HER2 positive breast cancer. No other metastases were found in bones or other organs.

Exemestane and Herceptin were started in June 2014, and she is now over seven years in remission after triple-positive breast treated cancer solely with antihormonal therapy and Herceptin.

Take home messages for all three women in this chapter will appear at the end of the chapter.

Gloria's Story

In November 2003, cancer knocked on my door. I noticed shooting pain in my right breast that would come and go. Then, I found a lump. I immediately made an appointment with my doctor who, in turn, ordered a biopsy. The diagnosis came back: breast cancer. Cancer? What was that? Why me? That night, my husband and I sat down to make arrangements as we figured I would be first to leave this world. Done in by cancer? This was a challenge, and we were going to face it head-on. I was fifty-three years old and had a wonderful husband and daughter. I was working for an airline, which allowed my husband and I to travel at any time. Life was good.

In December, my husband and I met with the surgeon. I thought that I could save the breast and scheduled a lumpectomy. It was later determined that I needed to have the breast removed. A mastectomy was performed on April 4, 2004, and a regimen of chemotherapy followed thereafter.

Before I started my chemo, an appointment was set up for me to visit the chemotherapy area to get acquainted with the nurses and to learn what to expect in each session. I remember calling my nurse before the first session and asking, "Do you think I'll lose my hair?" and her response was, "Gloria, you have not accepted the fact that you will be losing your hair, and it will be after your first chemo treatment." Sure enough, being as vain as any woman, the shock of finding gobs of hair on my pillow and coming out by the handfuls was tough. Once I finished with the chemo regimen, it was recommended to proceed with Herceptin. Through all this, my husband, daughter, family, and friends were by my side. I cannot imagine what I would have done if I had to embark on this journey alone. After the Herceptin infusions were complete, I continued to see my oncologist every three months, tapering to every six months as my markers were normal. Ultimately, I no longer had to see my oncologist. Everything was good, and life was rosy.

I did well for ten years and thought that, surely, I'd beaten cancer. Life was going well. In 2014, I went for my yearly gynecologic checkup and found that my fibroids had grown, and the doctor suggested I have them removed. I was not experiencing any symptoms, so I was less enthusiastic about removal. My doctor stated, "If they should burst, you are to seek treatment immediately." Hmmm. My daughter and I had planned a trip to London in two months, and this made me reconsider my options. All I could think about was, "What if I have an issue in London? Will my insurance cover me there? What if I die there?" I made my decision and called my doctor, who immediately scheduled the procedure. The surgeon found the fibroids to be too large for laparoscopic removal, and a laparotomy was necessary. Breast cancer cells were found in an ovary; and a, a hysterectomy was performed. At that time, it was suggested that I see an oncologist for further treatment.

That's when Dr. Vogel entered my life. My daughter and I met with him to explain my situation, and he suggested that I start a regimen of Herceptin. That was in 2014, and I have received an infusion every three weeks since that time. It's been said that Herceptin is a miracle drug, and I definitely feel this way. I'm still here. I'm proof that there is life after being diagnosed with HER2 positive, stage 4 breast cancer. I feel terrific, my life is good, and I have no complaints. I have been blessed with the best family, friends, and medical staff. What more could I ask for? I cherish every day and make the most of each day, as I know the precious value of life. I appreciate the small things and remind myself every day to stay strong. Life is to be lived, and I am excited to see where it takes me.

2: Terrie

Terrie, at age forty-four, was diagnosed with a large tumor in the left breast in 1994. She was treated with chemotherapy followed by left breast lumpectomy for infiltrating ductal carcinoma with two positive nodes.

She received Cytoxan, methotrexate, and 5 fluorouracil chemotherapy (CMF) after the surgical procedure. This was followed by radiation and five years of tamoxifen.

In December 2005, Terrie developed gynecologic bleeding that was noted to be related to an ovarian recurrence of breast cancer. She underwent removal of her uterus, fallopian tubes, and ovaries. The tumor was ER positive and HER2 negative.

She has been on letrozole therapy since December 2005 with no evidence of recurrence. She has experienced issues with lymphedema and recurrent cellulitis of the left arm requiring regular lymphedema treatment.

She also has osteoporosis. Various therapies have been offered, but Terrie has declined.

As of June 2020, Terrie is fifteen years disease-free on letrozole after ovarian recurrence.

Terrie's Story

It was June of 1994, and I had just turned forty-four. I was entering a time of new beginnings, and I was excited about the possibilities that lay before me. Just a month earlier, I left a long-tenured job to build a business on my own. I already had two signed contracts, one of which involved spending three weeks in the Berkshires, and I couldn't wait to leave. Before I did, though, I had my annual mammogram scheduled. When I went for the exam, the technician, (who ended up conducting my mammograms for the next twenty-five years until she retired), immediately noticed a flat area on the side of my left breast. She told me that she did not like the look of that area. She called the radiologist to ask that he be available to review the films. She took the expected images along with a few extra and sent me on my way. As I walked back into my office, which was only five minutes from the hospital, the phone was ringing. It was my gynecologist, who informed me that the radiologist found a suspicious area on the films and that she wanted me to consult with a surgeon immediately. Thus, began my journey.

My gynecologist, arranged for a visit with a surgeon within a day. I had met him two years before when I had a dense area in my breast that the gynecologist wanted to be sure wasn't hiding a potential cancer. At the time, it was determined to be loose and disorganized calcifications. The surgeon previously equated them to tropical depressions, which, while they have the potential to develop into hurricanes, might just as likely dissipate. We were going to watch it, but I conveniently put it out of my mind. I hadn't gone back. In hindsight, I should have returned.

The appointment with the surgeon was on a Friday afternoon. He called over to the hospital and asked if a pathologist would be available to review a biopsy before the end of the day. He did not want me facing the weekend without an answer. The results returned quickly, and I learned that I did indeed have breast cancer. He told me that while I could go anywhere in the world for treatment, if I wanted to stay local where I had a support system, he would get me into one of the best oncologists I'd find anywhere, Dr. Charles Vogel.

A series of tests revealed several types of breast cancer intertwined. It was noted to be an orange-sized tumor. Best practice dictated a mastectomy. I was only forty-four and single. Keeping my breast was of paramount importance to me. Dr. Vogel started me on a strong regimen of chemotherapy prior to surgery in an attempt to reduce the tumor size, and it worked to a degree. While the surgeon made no promises, he ultimately was able to respect my wishes and preserve the breast. I followed the surgery with another round of chemotherapy and radiation, which, with Dr. Vogel's blessing, was given together. I wanted this experience behind me.

Other than the development of lymphedema, which cropped up immediately, for eleven years, the experience *was* behind me. Then, I experienced breakthrough bleeding. I had gone into chemo-induced menopause after my second treatment, so I knew something was wrong. A scan revealed a tumor on my left ovary. It was diagnosed as a metastasis of the breast cancer. I was referred to a gynecological oncologist. He performed a radical hysterectomy, which, fortunately, required no follow-up with either chemotherapy or radiation. Five weeks later, I was on a long-scheduled family trip to Chile, confident that this was all behind me once and for all.

I remain confident all these years later.

Throughout my experiences with breast cancer, people have often commented on how calmly and gracefully I dealt with the disease. They all hypothesized that I must have done my share of crying in private. While I know that would have been understandable, I never did. Nor did I ever ask, "Why me?" Nobody goes through life unscathed. This was my lot. I felt it was better than what many others confront.

I am lucky. Every one of my doctors was extraordinary. I was also born with rose-colored glasses firmly planted on my face. I am not a person who buys trouble. If I am faced with a problem, I will confront it squarely. I never waste time and effort worrying about something that might never happen. This inborn personality trait was invaluable as I made my journey. I also credit gathering with friends who were also facing challenges to meditate on a regular basis, receiving massages throughout, and continuing to work. Though I never made that original trip to the Berkshires, I was working in the Bahamas eight days after my original surgery. Continuing to live life throughout my treatments made a big difference for me.

So much is known about breast cancer today. So many more treatments are available. The doctors and nurses of the oncology world are a special breed. I have found that putting trust in the science and the people and letting go with what we cannot control makes the burden of this scary diagnosis easier to carry.

My surgeon once told me my treatment would take about six months. I responded that I would give him six months to "fix me," and I started the clock. I was convinced that I would, in fact, be "fixed" within that timeframe. It took a bit longer, and of course, I had the second bout. But in the grand scheme of things, an extra couple of months is worth the twenty-six years I've enjoyed so far and the many more I still expect to enjoy.

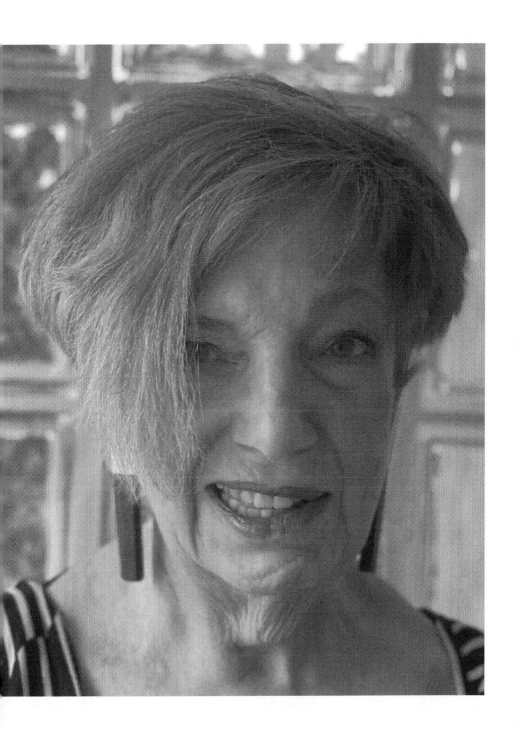

3: Barbara

Barbara presented with a tumor of the ovary in 1999 with right-sided lobular carcinoma of the breast diagnosed concurrently (de novo stage IV disease).

Her breast tumor was treated with lumpectomy without radiation or axillary dissection, as she already have metastatic disease.

After removal of the ovaries, which confirmed MBC, she received tamoxifen and had a response lasting over *ten* years. During that time, she moved from New York to Florida

Over the next seventeen to eighteen years, Barbara was treated mostly with antihormonal therapies at the time of each disease recurrence as noted below.

After progression on tamoxifen, it was stopped, a strategy called tamoxifen withdrawal, and that lasted for a year. She then received anastrozole, then anastrozole withdrawal, followed by Faslodex, and then Faslodex plus Ibrance. When she was diagnosed with bone metastases in 2016, she started Xgeva.

At one of her relapses, she enrolled on a clinical trial of enobosarm, a nonvirilizing androgen male hormone. This is an investigational drug that shows promise in ER-positive patients. She took this drug from November 2016, to February 2017, but derived no benefit.

She then received Doxil (stealth liposomal doxorubicin). Doxil is a much better tolerated form of Adriamycin. She discontinued that medication due to a severe skin reaction.

Multiple urinary tract infections led to a diagnosis of biopsy proven metastatic disease to the bladder. This caused bilateral obstructions and required bilateral stent placement.

Xeloda was started in May 2017, and her tumor markers dropped dramatically. She felt well, and at repeat cystoscopy, her bladder tumor was no longer present.

Unfortunately, in August 2018, Barbara was found to have disease intra-abdominally and in the liver. She started Abraxane with some improvement as of November 2018. About a week later, however, she had intestinal obstruction from intra-abdominal tumors, finally passing December 4, 2018, after having MBC for *twenty* years.

Barbara's Story

In 1999, my wife (Barbara) was diagnosed with metastatic breast cancer, which was originally found on her ovary. We received conflicting treatment recommendations from her breast surgeon and her oncologist. We went to Memorial Sloan Kettering for another opinion. This doctor agreed with the less-aggressive approach of Barbara's oncologist and almost, more importantly, advised Barbara not to "give away her jewelry" quite yet. She was right for almost twenty years. In 2001, we retired to Florida although Barbara was only fifty-eight and I was sixty. We wanted to spend whatever time we had left together. Over the ensuing years, both our daughters were married, two grandsons were born, and we grew even closer. We traveled many times to see our daughters and their families up north. We also visited our son, first in Buffalo and then in Colorado, when he relocated. We made many new friends. We were able to travel often, within the US, Canada, and to Europe, Israel, China, South America, and the Caribbean. We generally enjoyed life.

Barbara's tamoxifen treatment stopped working after about eleven years, and our doctor's visits became more stressful, while awaiting tumor marker numbers and scan results. During one particular visit, Barbara only wanted to know if she would make it to our eldest grandson's Bar Mitzvah. She did. During most of Barbara's treatment, she was asymptomatic. Although we had to cancel some trips (not all) because of newly diagnosed tumors, she felt pretty well. In fact, she often said that I was more stressed than she while awaiting test results. Almost twenty years later, December 2018, my girls, in-between tears, sorted through Barbara's jewelry. I miss her. We all do.

1–3, Gloria, Terrie, and Barbara: Takeaway

The three patients in this chapter shared the common presentation of ovarian metastases and all experienced protracted periods of disease control. They also shared the common denominator of ER positivity. As the reader shall see in later chapters, (especially chapter 5), some women with ER positive tumors can have very protracted clinical courses. In this chapter, Barb exemplifies a protracted clinical course. So, whether presentation with an ovarian metastases may portend a better, longer term clinical course remains speculative. Gloria had a HER2 positive tumor and remains on an aromatase inhibitor (AI, an antihormonal therapy) as well as Herceptin. Terrie has remained on an AI alone after surgery for fifteen-plus years.

Barbara lived for twenty years after the diagnosis of her ovarian metastases. She had excellent disease control on tamoxifen alone after surgery for ten years and remained on antihormonal treatments for another seven years prior to treatment with chemotherapy before finally succumbing to her disease. For the first eighteen years of her clinical course, Barbara and her husband, Bob, lived reasonably normal, happy, and fruitful lives, enjoying wonderful travel experiences in the US and abroad. Barb's tumor remained hormonally sensitive for a long period of time just as the women in chapter 5.

CHAPTER V

Hormone Receptor Positive HER2 Negative

Prolonged Hormonal Responsiveness

Introduction

This chapter deals with the most common breast cancer subtype, which constitutes 70% of all patients. Using genomic testing such as MammaPrint, NanoString, and others, these tumors are further subdivided into luminal A and luminal B. Luminal A tumors tend to grow more slowly and have a better prognosis than luminal B tumors, even when these patients develop metastatic disease. The other two intrinsic subtypes using genomic testing are HER2 positive and triple negative (negative for ER, PR, and HER2).

Fortunately, we have many antihormonal therapies that can be used to relieve symptoms and prolong life in ER positive breast cancer. These include, but are not limited to, removal of the ovaries in premenopausal patients; Zoladex and Lupron to shut down the ovaries in premenopausal patients; tamoxifen, which is largely used today in premenopausal patients, but is also highly effective in postmenopausal patients; toremifene (very similar to tamoxifen, but FDA approved only for postmenopausal patients). The data are too limited for the FDA to approve it in premenopausal women, though it is widely used in that subset of women (23). In postmenopausal patients, aromatase inhibitors (anastrozole, letrozole, exemestane) and fulvestrant, a selective estrogen receptor down regulator (SERD) are commonly used. Although not often used these days, progestins like megestrol acetate (Megace) and, strangely enough, high-dose estrogen (24, 25) have been able to induce remission in some patients. As of 2020, the antihormonal field has been revolutionized as we have discovered targeted drugs that potentiate the action of antihormonal therapy. The first in use was the MTOR inhibitor everolimus (26) and, more recently, the CDK4/6 inhibitors palbociclib (Ibrance), ribociclib (Kisqali), and abamaciclib (Verzenio). These latter drugs are now virtually routinely used with an antihormone agent as the first treatment for ER positive/HER2 negative MBC. Studies in early-stage ER positive, HER2 positive patients are in progress with the CDK4/6 inhibitors, and the 2020s will be the decade of discovery as many targeted agents are under study, as are several oral SERDs (selective estrogen receptor down regulator), which will try to challenge the injectable fulvestrant as the dominant SERD. I remain optimistic that enobosarm, a nonvirilizing androgen, will ultimately give us another hormonal option. Male hormones were used in MBC in the 1960s and 1970s, but rarely today.

1: Carol

Carol developed a right breast cancer in 1990 at age sixty-one with two positive lymph nodes. She underwent mastectomy and implant reconstruction. Her tumor was found to be ER positive, PR positive, and HER2 unknown, as HER2 testing was not universal in the early 1990s.

She received adjuvant CMF chemotherapy from September 1990 to March 1991 and was on tamoxifen from 1991 to 1993.

Carol developed a chest wall recurrence in February 2000, about ten years after her original diagnosis. Her implant and recurrence were removed. Subsequently, she received radiation followed by Taxotere and vinorelbine (Navelbine) with extreme toxicity. At this point, she transferred her medical care to our practice.

She was first placed on tamoxifen rechallenge and received that drug from 2000 to May 2004 with good response. This demonstrated that although one has received tamoxifen in the past, they can still respond to tamoxifen for metastatic disease.

At tamoxifen relapse, she received Aromasin from May 2004 to August 2004, when it was was discontinued secondary to weight gain and joint pain.

The initial trial of aggressive chemotherapy and the subsequent hormonal treatments were given in an attempt to avoid another recurrence. Thus, the patient was treated at that time as stage 4 NED (see chapter 3 after local regional recurrence).

In spite of the treatment, she developed disease in the bones in July 2008, and anastrozole was started with Zometa shortly after. The lesions resolved nicely on this therapy, and she has remained on anastrozole for the past eleven years.

She underwent an aortic valve replacement in 2009. She also had removal of a right arm melanoma removed in 2010 or 2011.

As of July 2021, she has no evidence of recurrence on her first hormonal therapy for systemic metastatic disease to bone. It has been nineteen years since her first recurrence on the chest wall and twelve years since her relapse in bone.

1, Carol: Takeaway

It is a misconception that just because the patient has a mastectomy cancer cannot recur where the breast mass was removed. Carol had a relapse in her skin at the site where the breast had been removed; this is called a chest wall relapse. Management of these tumors remains controversial in 2020. The likelihood of recurrence ultimately in other areas is high (chapter 3: "Stage IV NED"). If the tumor is estrogen-receptor positive, removal of the tumor, radiation, and antihormonal therapy is indicated. It remains unclear what the role of chemotherapy is in ER positive patients with local-regional recurrence. No controlled and randomized trials have successfully addressed this question. Even in the CALOR trial as discussed in chapter 3, while in ER negative patients, there is a 10% benefit for chemotherapy added to surgical removal and radiation, results for hormone receptor positive patients did not show a statistically significant benefit for chemotherapy (17).

Assuming that Carol's chest wall recurrence was the start of her metastatic process, she is alive nineteen years after that recurrence (as some chest wall recurrences can be cured with surgery, radiation, and hormonal therapy). Her survival without recurrence from the diagnosis of bone metastases has been twelve years on the first and only treatment she has received to date for metastases to a distant site (bone). The median time to relapse for a large series of patients on first line anastrozole for MBC is fourteen to sixteen months. Carol's eleven-year response, while extraordinary, is not too different from other patients mentioned in this chapter.

Carol's doctors in the year 2000, possibly following some of the publications from the MD Cancer Center (18), treated her with chemotherapy after radiation and before hormonal therapy. Unfortunately, the toxicity was excessive, and she was hospitalized for complications. As of 2019, it remains controversial as to whether chemotherapy should be used sequentially with hormonal therapy in patients with ER positive local recurrences.

My Journey with the Big *C*—Cancer—
Breast Cancer: Carol's Story

August 1990. It all started with a shower. I felt a lump … what could that be? I just had a mammogram a month prior, but I did start on estrogen three months before that. Could estrogen be involved? Better call my gynecologist and see what he thinks. Within a week, I was scheduled for a mastectomy. Hindsight says "Slow down, talk to others, do some research, don't rush into major decisions unless it is an emergency." However, that day in the shower started my journey with the big *C*—breast cancer—and it will be a part of my life until I am gone.

The cancer was an infiltrating ductal carcinoma, which invaded two lymph nodes out of twelve and estrogen receptor positive. I researched and talked with other doctors and knowledgeable friends and chose my oncologist carefully. I was recommended to have chemotherapy. Chemotherapy was scheduled—6 sessions of CMF (Cytoxan, methotrexate, 5-FU) starting in September 1990. I have to admit, I was very scared not knowing what to expect—throw up on the spot, get dizzy, pass out? The doctor said I needed to stay away from people, especially if my blood count was low. Perhaps I should stop working. I was the director of the largest concert series hosted in a church in the United States. I had about twenty-six performances that year, and I loved what I was doing. I gave it much thought and discussed it with John, my husband, and I decided not to stay home and "babysit" my cancer, but to work every day. I did work every day and never missed a concert. When my count was low, the women in my office protected me from seeing anyone, and I was very careful and did not get sick. I lost a lot of weight, had terrible mouth sores, was very tired most of the time, *but* I did everything that I needed to do when it had to be done. I had many people praying for me, and God gave me the strength and determination to work.

What I have learned about myself is that, initially, I may react to terrible news or circumstances, but after I get over the initial shock, my mind takes over. God has given me the gift of being able to handle things pretty well and to even take charge of events in my life when possible. Cancer is huge and very frightening, but I was determined not to let it control my life.

After my treatments, I had a great desire to go back to teaching elementary school gifted kids, where I felt I could make a difference in their lives. I didn't know why or how, because I had never planned to go back to teaching, and I loved what I was doing with the concerts. However, in 1993, I followed my heart, retired from the music job, and went back teaching grades 2 to 5 with gifted children in Sunrise, Florida. I absolutely loved it. Soon, a new challenge …

In September 1993, my son Brad was diagnosed with a brain tumor—a glioblastoma multiforme. He was given three months to live, but he announced to me that he would live to know his child (wife, Krissy, was pregnant). He lived one year and one day, and his older daughter was age five years and his baby was six months when he died (October 19, 1994). Because of my experience with cancer, he was open to wanting me to go with him for his treatments (chemo/radiation) and tests. He talked with me about how he felt and dealt with what was happening. He also worked every day and helped at the cancer institute talking with and encouraging others with cancer. One day I said to him, "Brad, I don't know how you are handing all of this." He looked at me and said, *"Mom, I watched you do it."* At that point, I was able to thank God for my cancer because it opened a door for me to be able to help my son, Brad, live through his cancer.

Another challenge … January 2000, I found *another* mass in the same breast. A biopsy proved that the mass was positive for breast cancer and extended to all the margins, including the capsule of the implant that had been put in after my first cancer surgery in 1990. On February 8, a mastectomy was performed to remove the capsule and implant. My cancer was estrogen- and progesterone-receptor positive and negative for P53 and HER2/neu. I met with my oncologist, and he strongly suggested treatment with Taxotere and Navelbine, but for only three sessions, which would be followed by twenty-eight sessions of radiation therapy.

At that point, I decided that I wanted to take my gifted children at school on this new cancer journey with me. I felt that in their lifetime, they would have to deal with cancer personally or through their family or friends, and I wanted them to see how someone could handle it with humor, education, faith, and guts. My two principals and parents *agreed to trust me.* I decided the students and I would write a little booklet about our experiences—to document everything they learned and everything we did. To introduce my cancer to my students, my daughter-in-law gave me a CD with the music "Don't worry about a thing … everything is gonna turn out all right." I told the students that I would be out of school for a week because I had a growth in my chest, and it had to be taken out but that I was not worried, and I didn't want them to be worried, so we then did a conga line around the room, listening to the tape and singing.

When I came back to school after the surgery, I brought an *oncology nurse* (who was one of my parents) to talk to the children about the words *cancer, chemotherapy, radiation*, and what it all meant. I explained that I would lose my hair with the chemotherapy, and I wanted their opinion on what color and style wig I should have. So they took a photo of my face, put it in the computer, and started putting different hairdos and colors on my face. After a couple weeks of chemo, I told them that, on Monday, my hair would be gone and that I would wear my new wig and that they would absolutely *love it*. Well, on Monday, I wore a wig of long brown dreadlocks, and the kids, well, some were polite and told me I looked beautiful; but some of the honest ones said, "You are kidding, right?" It was such fun, and I had to finally confess that it wasn't really my wig. I told them that every couple weeks, we would have a bad hair day, and who knew what I would show up in? I emailed all my teacher friends and asked them to send me ridiculous wigs to wear, and we had several bad hair days.

When I was ready to begin the radiation, we had a field trip to the hospital to see what that machine would look like and to talk with the radiation oncologist. One of my very talented gifted kids asked, "Are you going to glow in the dark?" He suggested they could make a science fair project out of me. They all laughed, and I said, "Well, I don't know. We will have to check it out after I begin my treatments."

On a Friday, I told the students that I was starting my radiation on Monday, so on Wednesday, we would see if I was glowing in the dark. Monday and Tuesday, they were so excited and hardly could wait until Wednesday. This is what I did: I put a green glow stick in the pocket of my blouse and closed a suit jacket over it. I took the students into a room where there were no windows and closed the door and slowly opened the jacket, so the glow stick glowed a green color coming from my chest. I still laugh thinking about it. The students screamed in excitement. Of course, in a couple minutes, I had to tell them the truth, and then we had a little lesson on what radiation really does to the body.

As all these things were happening, we were writing them down and illustrating our booklet called "Cancer + Humor = Understanding." What did the children learn? Here are some of the things the students wrote in the booklet: "Cancer is not contagious, and you can't catch it"; "Don't be afraid of cancer but learn all you can about the disease"; "Laugh, laugh, and laugh"; "You can have fun even if you have cancer"; "Your attitude will help you go through it"; "Get the best treatment"; "There are side effects with chemo, and radiation"; "Have a healthy respect for it"; "Research and learn all you can"; "Love each other just the same"; "Take care of yourself and your body"; and much more. After this was all over, I wrote for a grant and had the booklet copied and put into every school library in Broward County. I would have loved to have had it published to go into oncology offices, but I never pursued that idea.

Two of my grandchildren attended the school that I taught in when I had my cancer, and they rode home from school with me on Fridays. They were always bugging me to see me without hair, but I wasn't comfortable with that idea. One day, my five-year-old granddaughter said with her hands on her hips, "Nana, what difference does it make? You are still just our Nana," so the wig came off. They rubbed my head, and we laughed, and I put it back on, and that was that! Out of the mouth of babes.

Yes, I lost my breast and my hair, but not my determination, my courage, my humor, my love. I am still just Nana—Grandma, sis, mom, Carol!

Is my cancer over? Well, July 2008, it had returned in my bones with Dr. Vogel as my oncologist. I was on Zometa for a couple years and started on Arimidex, which I am still on, and he is amazed that it is now 2020 and that drug continues to be effective, and the cancer is still under control! I am now eighty-two years old, and breast cancer has been a part of my life for thirty years! I mostly ignore the possibility of more cancer except when I have a PET/CT scan or the CA15-3 bloodwork checked every three to six months. It is no longer *when* but *if* it returns, and I am pretty convinced it won't pay another visit.

My cancer over the years has opened many doors for me to share, help, and encourage others, as well as helping some friends prepare for dying. I do thank God for my cancer and the opportunities that it has given me. My cancer helped my son, my students, my grandchildren, and it made me a better person—more caring about others. I have found joy in my life in spite of the circumstances … not always happiness, but always *joy*. Life is a precious gift, and I value each day! Every night when I get into bed I say, "Thank you, God, for another day."

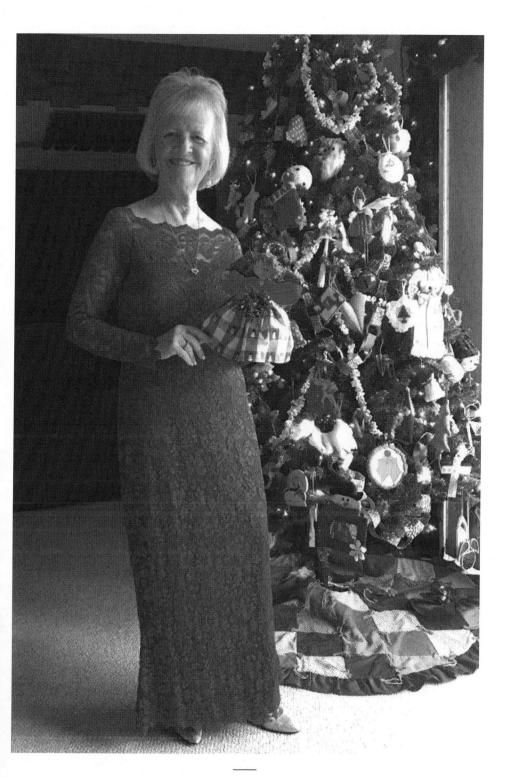

2: Patrice

Patrice was diagnosed with breast cancer with one of eleven lymph nodes positive at age thirty-five in December of 2000. She underwent bilateral mastectomies with reconstruction. The tumor was ER positive and PR positive HER2 3+ positive. This was in the pre-adjuvant Herceptin era, and the 3+ may have been a false positive assay, as we still see many false positives even in 2020.

She received adjuvant therapy with AC ×4 followed by Taxotere ×4, and then took tamoxifen.

In March 2003, there was suspicion of metastasis in the sacrum, but no biopsy was performed. She was given Zoladex to suppress her ovarian function, plus anastrozole, and was enrolled in a clinical trial of a therapeutic vaccine. Letrozole was substituted for anastrozole after musculoskeletal complaints while on anastrozole.

In May 2003, radiation was given to the solitary bone metastasis in the sacrum.

She continued on Zoladex and letrozole until 2014 when there was slow increase of cancer markers leading to a metastatic workup, which identified three new bone lesions.

As there was progression in bone, she was taken off letrozole. However, she continued on Zoladex, and started on fulvestrant (Faslodex) after eleven years on the previous regimen.

In order to stop Zoladex, she elected to have removal of her uterus, fallopian tubes, and ovaries, which was performed on December 24, 2014. She then continued on fulvestrant until January 2017, when progression of MBC was demonstrated after two and a half years on this drug.

Between 2017 and March 2021, Patrice received multiple systemic therapies including tamoxifen and Ibrance, Xeloda, Navelbine and Xeloda, letrozole and Verzenio, Abraxane, Gemzar, IMMU-132, and eribulin. However, in March 2021, her liver size increased, and she felt ill. Treatment was unsuccessfully changed back to Abraxane. Unfortunately, after eighteen years of MBC, Patrice's liver metastases had progressed to a point where hospice was recommended, and she left all who loved her on April 23, 2021

2, Patrice: Takeaway

Like Carol, Patrice had a very long duration of response to hormonal therapy as a solo treatment for her bone-only metastatic disease. Although premenopausal at diagnosis of her bone metastasis, she was rendered postmenopausal medically and treated with letrozole, a drug only effective in postmenopausal women. Carole received anastrozole, but two other drugs, letrozole and exemestane, are similar and called aromatase inhibitors (AI). These only work in postmenopausal women as their mechanism of action is to stop the tiny amounts of estrogen produced at that time. Since the postmenopausal ovary does not produce estrogen, it is produced indirectly by the adrenal glands. These little glands, which sit on top of the kidney, produce male hormones (testosterone) that are converted by an enzyme aromatase, most of which occurs in fatty tissue. These three aromatase inhibitors antagonize the enzyme aromatase, preventing estrogen production. Perhaps because Patrice was thin with limited fatty tissue, there was less aromatase to antagonize, leading to a longer response. However, this is only speculation. In order for Patrice to benefit from an AI as a premenopausal woman, it was necessary to suppress her ovarian function. Initially, this was done with Zoladex and later with removal of the ovaries. Patrice lived eighteen years with MBC, with excellent quality of life until the last few months.

Patrice's Story

My name is Patrice. I have officially been living with breast cancer since November 28, 2000. My story begins in July of 1999. I was thirty-five then, happily married for ten years with two children—Mallorie, age 5, and Rachel, age 2. My life was good, though sometimes hectic. However, behind the scenes, I had been noticing that my right nipple was inverting. I also noticed a crusty discharge on the nipple. I thought nothing of these changes taking place. I was not aware that these findings could be possible signs of breast cancer. However, my girlfriend was diagnosed with breast cancer, and this prompted me to begin performing self-breast exams when in the shower. This is how I found a mass in my right breast.

I made an appointment with my gynecologist to confirm my finding. I then underwent my first mammogram, which showed "no suspicious mass or calcification." A follow-up mammogram was recommended at age forty unless something should change. My gynecologist continued to monitor me. It was not until the early part of 2000 that I had an ultrasound that confirmed a solid nodule. A biopsy was recommended. The pathology returned with "no evidence of malignancy" with a recommendation for a six-month sonographic follow-up. In October of 2000, I underwent a follow-up ultrasound, which showed enlargement of the mass. An excisional biopsy was recommended. I was worried and starting to feel afraid. I was referred to a surgeon who performed an incisional biopsy to remove the mass in November of 2000 right after Thanksgiving. My husband and I met with the surgeon to review the findings. I still can remember this moment vividly. We waited a very long time in a full waiting room and then for a long time in the exam room. I was sitting on the exam table in a gown when the doctor finally entered the room. He had my file open in his hand. He told us that I had cancer. It was at that moment that I stopped hearing what was being said. I looked at my husband and noticed his entire facial expression shift to visible shock. I remember reassuring him that I would be OK. The tumor was found to contain both ductal and lobular cancer without clear margins. The doctor left to find the name of a specialist. We waited again for some time, but he never returned. He was so busy. Finally, a nurse entered to say that I could get dressed and check out. My husband hugged me and tried to reassure me that everything would be fine. I knew that I was going into this with a loving and supportive husband and family, which was a great comfort. My drive home was full of tears. We were in separate cars. We spoke on the phone to each other and discussed what was next and how to tell our children. I remember the song on the radio playing "The Great Beyond" by R.E.M. It is a song about attempting the impossible. To this day, I still cry when I hear this song

I found a breast surgeon and a plastic surgeon and was scheduled for a bilateral mastectomy with reconstruction. However, three days prior to the procedure, I was notified that my father, who lived a couple hours away, was very ill in the hospital. I caught a flight that day to see him and say goodbye. The next day, my sister Marsha and I drove back to my home. Marsha was going to help with our children. On December 21, I underwent a bilateral mastectomy with reconstruction. The left breast was removed prophylactically. This was the same day my father passed away.

My cancer was ER and PR positive, but HER2 negative. I met with a few oncologists for recommendations on a plan of treatment. Thankfully, I decided upon Dr. Vogel. I refused to read or hear about any statistics. I did not want to know what my odds were for dying. I was just happy to be alive and have a treatment available. There was great optimism all around me. On February 2, 2001, I signed on to take part in a phase III study. I remember the first day of my chemo. The nurses and office staff were so kind and loving. My husband was by my side. By the fourth treatment, my hair was coming out. I was hoping that I would still have hair for my father's memorial. I did. Ultimately, I had a head-shaving event at my sister's house with my two children and husband. We tried to keep it upbeat and fun as my children were there. My brother, who was bald, was also there. My brother and I took pictures together. Now we really looked alike! I had my eighth and final dose of chemo on July 3, 2001. My children and I made a cake to celebrate. "No More Chemo" was written on it in red frosting, which matched my red bandana.

On September 11, 2001, I underwent an operation to replace the breast expanders with saline implants and have my port removed. It was during my surgery that our world as we knew it was changed forever. As I was coming out of anesthesia, a nurse told me something horrible had happened. I thought she was talking about me and my surgery. A wave of panic washed through my mind. The nurse then told me how a plane had crashed into the World Trade Center. Later, as I lay on the moving stretcher on the way to my room, I asked my husband if a plane really crashed into the World Trade Center. I don't even remember his answer. My hospital bed mate, who was a local gynecologist, spent the evening trying to contact her sister who worked in one of the towers.

I was recommended to take tamoxifen for the next five years, which was the current standard post-treatment. The chemo treatment room, the patients, the nurses, and the staff all had become my safety shield. The thought of recurrence was a constant in the back of my mind. I was blessed that I was doing well and started to get on with my life of being a mom and wife. My husband and I started a workout challenge, and I had my twenty-year high school reunion to attend. There were birthday parties and dance recitals. I had started to notice an achy pain in my left tailbone area. On March 27, 2001, a scan confirmed that the cancer had progressed. Hello, metastatic breast cancer. I was now stage IV. I was not interested in hearing about any of the statistics associated with MBC. My husband and

I met with Dr. Vogel to work out a new plan of treatment, and my husband asked about my prognosis. I stopped the conversation and told them both that I did not want to know. Once we had a plan in place, I left my husband behind to talk to Dr. Vogel. When he came out of his office, his face was gray, and once again, that look of doom had overcome his normal cheery disposition. He gave me a big hug, and I began treatment. The plan was to have a monthly shot of Zoladex in my abdomen to put me into menopause and to take Femara, which has a hormone therapy drug. This treatment plan qualified me to take part in a study for the Theratope vaccine, which was an immune therapy. I had monthly injections in each thigh. I also underwent radiation to the painful area, which gave me relief. I was closely monitored at regular doctor visits and with imaging. These drugs kept me stable until late 2010 (about nine years) and I continued to move forward in my life with a positive attitude. It was not until I became more active in online MBC groups that I really became aware of the terrible statistics for people with MBC. Through these groups, I have made many friends, and I have seen many perish. I have become more vocal about the importance of research. I have had more radiation since then, been on more drugs, and have lost my hair a couple more times. I do not let this disease define me or scare me. My goal is to live my life and be a strong role model for my children. I believe I have accomplished this. I have learned how to overcome the disappointment of each progression. Here I am, still alive in 2020. I have been thriving for twenty years and metastatic for seventeen. I have experienced many milestones. My life is good; I am happy and still happily married to my husband, who supports me in every way possible. Our children are now twenty-three and twenty-six.

3: Roz

In 1993, at age forty-seven, Roz underwent a right mastectomy for lobular invasive carcinoma. She developed chest wall recurrence in 1996 and was treated with CAF chemotherapy (Cytoxan, Adriamycin, 5-fluorouracil) and then took anastrozole for about twelve years in the stage IV NED situation (see chapter 3, "Stage IV NED").

About twelve years after her chest wall recurrence, Roz relapsed in bone in 2009.

Her treatment has been as follows:

- October 2009–March 2011: Exemestane (Aromasin).
- March 2011—April 2012: Faslodex (fulvestrant).
- April 2012—February 2015: Tamoxifen.
- February 2015—March 2016: Tamoxifen withdrawal. In a previous chapter, we have discussed tamoxifen withdrawal as a treatment. Roz had a thirteen-month response to that maneuver (see chapter 4, "Barbara"; chapter 5, "Mildred").
- May 2016—February 2017: Letrozole and Ibrance.
- February 2017—June 2017: Estrogen. Although her tumor markers started to go down, she found that estrogen side effects were intolerable secondary to vaginal bleeding.
- March 2017—September 2017: Estrogen withdrawal.
- September 2017—April 2018: Anastrozole and Faslodex.
- April 2018—August 2018: Tamoxifen and Afinitor.
- August 2018—October 2018: Tamoxifen withdrawal again.

In 2018, we tested the tissue specimen removed in 2012 at the time of posterior chest wall recurrence. Interestingly, it revealed a high mutational burden and could be predictive of a response to some type of immunotherapeutic manipulation. We also found the mutation PIK3CA, making her eligible to receive alpelisib (Piqray), a second line antagonist. In October 2019, she started fulvestrant with Piqray, but she discontinued treatment quickly in November 2019 due to severe rash and severe headaches.

In February 2020, she restarted a combination of anastrozole and fulvestrant, but after a few months, that too was found ineffective.

Over the years, Roz has lived a completely normal life and has never been in the hospital. When she developed bone metastasis in 2009, she was started on Zometa, which was exchanged for Xgeva in 2016. She is currently receiving this every three months.

As of September 2020, she started Megace, which continued as of December 2020. With markers continuing to rise on Megace, Piqray (predicted to be effective by next generation sequencing) was restarted at half dose with Megace. She is tolerating this dose well, does not yet need glucose-lowering agents, and her tumor markers are falling as of March 2021.

Roz has had metastatic disease for twenty-three years if one counts her chest wall recurrence as the start of her metastatic process. She has had systemic metastatic disease since 2009 and is thus eleven years with a diagnosis of systemic metastatic disease.

3, Roz: Takeaway

Roz has been dealing with metastatic disease for twenty-three years. This includes twelve years being disease-free after a chest wall recurrence and more than eleven years since the development of systemic (distant) metastases.

While most people think of chemotherapy (strong drugs) when they think of MBC, the real mainstay of treatment for patients with ER positive tumors is antihormonal therapy. Roz underwent fifteen forms of treatment since the diagnosis of a chest wall recurrence, and most of that time with reasonable disease control. She was also asymptomatic, with her treatment consisting of mostly anti hormonal therapy for twenty years before requiring a change in management to chemotherapy. Even during a brief course of chemotherapy, she had no symptoms secondary to that treatment, and when progression of disease was again noted, we returned to hormonal therapy.

Some of the treatments Roz received are of particular interest. She had almost three years of control on tamoxifen. Interestingly, patients with long periods of control on tamoxifen may respond to tamoxifen withdrawal (just stopping tamoxifen and adding nothing else). This was first shown by Tony Howell from Manchester, United Kingdom (27). He observed seventy-two such patients undergoing only tamoxifen withdrawal after first line tamoxifen therapy for MBC. Of those, 30% had a partial response or stable disease for a median duration of withdrawal response of ten months. Why should this be? Tamoxifen is a selective *estrogen receptor modulator* (SERM). This will act as an anti-estrogen on the tumor but as an estrogen on the bone (good effect) uterus (bad effect), and cholesterol (good effect). However, while it may suppress the tumor for long periods of time (see Barb, chapter 3), ultimately the estrogenic component of tamoxifen may take over and stimulate the tumor. Thus, stopping tamoxifen stops the stimulus, causing a tamoxifen withdrawal response. Roz had such a response for thirteen months, and Mildred (chapter 5) had a withdrawal response lasting seventeen months.

Another interesting treatment was the use of estradiol. Most people feel that estrogens stimulate breast cancer growth and virtually all our antitumor agents are aimed at reducing estrogen levels. However, estrogens were one of the only treatments for MBC prior to the discovery of tamoxifen in the mid-1970s. More recently, Dr. Mahtani and I published on this in 2009 (24), as did Dr. Matthew Ellis (25), who reported on a randomized trial of different doses. Roz's rising tumor markers rapidly decreased on this treatment. However, her course was complicated by uterine bleeding, which was too troublesome for her to continue. Regardless, the use of estrogen in some patients with refractory MBC can produce meaningful antitumor responses.

Finally, a PIK3CA mutation predicted the possible effectiveness of alpelisib (Piqray). While full dose of the drug produced intolerable toxicity, treatment at half dose months later appeared to be working in combination with Megace. In the twenty-first century, most physicians only think of Megace as an appetite stimulant. However, until the advent of the aromatase inhibitors, Megace was the first hormonal therapy used in MBC after progression on tamoxifen.

Mutation analysis also might predict for therapeutic activity for the immunotherapy agent Keytruda. While not currently necessary, this could be a consideration for Roz if Megace and Piqray stop working.

Roz's Story

Seventy-five years young and married for fifty-five years.

Today

I am a wife, mother of three married daughters and grandmother of seven. My life is busy with family, friends, golf, bridge, canasta, and mah-jongg. I've traveled extensively before COVID-19 and look forward to traveling in the future.

I have Metastatic Breast Cancer.

Yesterday

I was forty-eight years old and sitting in an oncologist's office in New York City when I was told that I had breast cancer and needed a mastectomy. I told the doctor that the tests were wrong because I felt well and could not comprehend that I had become a statistic. Clearly, I was wrong, and within a few weeks, I underwent a mastectomy, followed by nine months of intensive chemotherapy.

When I told my mother that I had finished my chemotherapy treatments and was ready to start to heal, she insisted that I go back to the oncologist and ask for radiation. So being afraid of both cancer and my mother, I went back to the medical oncologist and surgeon and asked them about radiation. They both said that there was nothing to radiate as the cancerous breast was removed. Unfortunately, my mother was right, as I had my first recurrence four and a half years later on the scar line from my mastectomy.

I underwent surgical resection of the tumor, and the surgeon found additional tumors on my chest. I then completed radiation and started a new medication called Arimidex. With Arimidex, I was recurrence-free for twelve years.

My next recurrence was in a bone called the iliac crest. At that time, I was put on Aromasin.

My next recurrence was a tumor in my back. A New York City hospital incorrectly diagnosed my tumor as nonmalignant. However, my tumor marker numbers were elevated, and Dr. Vogel ordered a biopsy, which showed that it was cancer. Dr. Vogel recommended a surgeon to remove the tumor. On removal, it was advanced and did not have clear margins. I then underwent radiation and was prescribed a new medication.

I am so grateful to Dr. Vogel for his care, his concern, and his knowledge. As the years pass, the cancer has spread to other bones, and I continue to try new therapies.

My mother encouraged me to take all of the recommended medications and treatments. She said that once I make a decision with the doctor, I should leave the office and try to forget that I have cancer and to live my life normally.

I've had several bumps (recurrences) in the road. I feel that I lead two lives: the happy one that I project to everyone and the other life filled with fear of the next recurrence.

Tomorrow

A new day! My thanks to Dr. Vogel and his staff for their concern, care, and professionalism. After eighteen years, I consider Dr. Vogel a friend. Every day, I hope for new treatments to be developed so that I can live the life my mother wanted for me.

4: Donald

Donald's history of breast cancer began in October 1997, at the age of sixty-seven. He underwent a right mastectomy, and his tumor was an ER positive and PR positve, infiltrating ductal carcinoma with fourteen of eighteen positive nodes. He was treated with AC chemotherapy followed by Taxotere and radiation therapy. He then took tamoxifen for two years followed by letrozole until 2008.

In November 2008, he developed a left breast cancer, and he underwent a left mastectomy with eighteen positive nodes. He was treated with Taxotere and Cytoxan for six doses followed by radiation.

In 2009, Donald began therapy with Lupron and tamoxifen. Therapy was continued until January 2014 when he was found to have metastatic disease. An elevated CEA led to the discovery of both bone metastasis and an enlarged left subclavicular mass (under the collarbone).

At this time, he was started on Xgeva to prevent skeletal-related fractures as related to bone metastases.

From 2014 to 2020, Donald received a number of systemic therapies including fulvestrant, fulvestrant and letrozole, metronomic methotrexate and cytoxan, Lupron and tamoxifen, exemestane and Ibrance, and Verzenio. In Though he progressed, there was a drop in tumor markers on Verzenio. November 2019, he started on eribulin, which continued until June 2020. He tried a lower dose that he was tolerating well. Unfortunately, in November 2020, he developed an unrelated gall bladder infection that led to multisystem organ failure, leading to his demise. It is ironic that after battling breast cancer for twenty-three years and MBC for six years that he would succumb to an unrelated medical issue at age ninety-one.

4, Donald: Takeaway

While there are approximately eight male breast cancer patients in my practice, only three men at the moment have MBC; one gentleman (Pedro) is early in the course with MBC and has had a nice response with tamoxifen. He is currently enjoying a symptom-free period of over one year on tamoxifen withdrawal (27).

Male breast cancer is a relatively rare disease, and every man with breast cancer should be tested for genetic mutations, as it is known that approximately 6% of men who are BRCA2 carriers will develop breast cancer by age seventy. In a study of 108 male breast cancer patients, 1.9% had a BRCA1 mutation and 7.4% had a BRCA2 mutation (28, 29). (Fortunately, Donald and Pedro are not gene carriers.) It is a misconception that these genetic defects can only be passed through the maternal bloodline. There are many families with genetic mutations that have started with the paternal bloodline.

Donald had locally advanced cancers of both his right and left breast which were diagnosed twenty-one years apart. Each was associated with numerous involved lymph nodes. He was appropriately treated for both of those tumors but ultimately developed MBC six years after the diagnosis of his second breast cancer. At age ninety-one, Donald remained very active with a shining personality and acerbic wit, always with a joke or two for his captive physician audience. Invariably accompanied by his wife, Irene, he faced his MBC and the treatment boldy and stoically. Every clinic appointment felt like a visit between friends rather than a professional interaction. Donald's disease was predominately in his bones, but he also had a large mass encroaching on his left shoulder. In the beginning, we joked about it interfering with his golf game (which he admitted was never so great to begin with). Realistically, however, it was ever so slowly limiting his range of motion in that arm.

Therapeutically, I cannot take much credit for finding drugs to slow down the progress of his cancer, as he did not gain a long period of disease control from any of the eight treatments he tried. Regardless, he remained in good spirits six years after the diagnosis of MBC. Unfortunately, his life was cut short, not by his MBC, but by an unrelated illness. RIP, old friend. I miss you and our visits together.

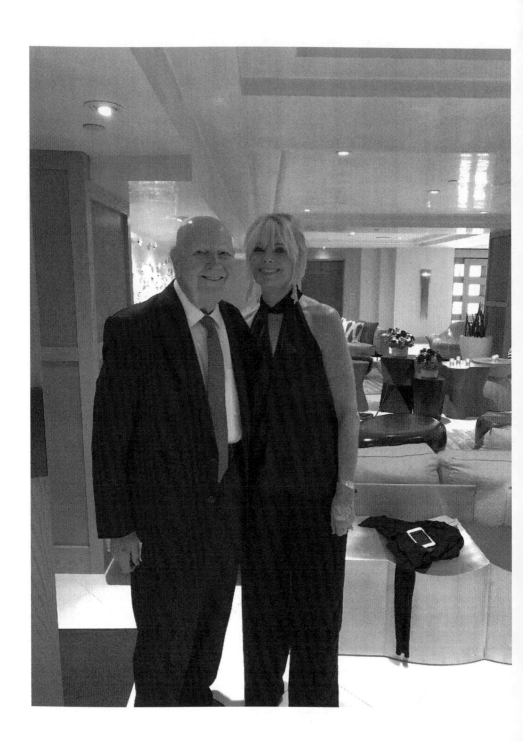

5: Judith

In February 2001, at the age of forty-seven, Judith had a right breast biopsy that diagnosed infiltrating ductal carcinoma associated with lobular carcinoma in situ.

She had a 1.7 cm tumor which was low grade, ER positive, and HER2 negative. An axillary dissection revealed two of ten positive nodes.

She completed Cytoxan, Adriamycin, fluorouracil chemotherapy, and radiation. Judith then took tamoxifen for eighteen months, which she stopped due to lack of insurance.

In October 2010, Judith had extensive skin lesions on the right breast, and she started letrozole. The response lasted for four years. She discontinued treatment due to unexpected sacral pain. When she stopped the letrozole, she stopped coming for follow-up visits

In May 2016, she returned and was noted to have bone metastasis, as well as the previously noted right breast skin lesions, which were relatively stable.

At that time, Judith started on enobosarm, which was available on a clinical trial. This drug is a nonvirilizing androgen (male hormone), but she did not respond and therefore stopped it in September 2016.

From September 2016 to July 2018, she took Ibrance and letrozole and experienced disease control for twenty-two months.

From August 2018 to November 2018, she took Faslodex but was noted to have progression.

Judith then began exemestane with Afinitor and responded well until January 2020 when, at progression, she began Verzenio with continuation of exemestane.

At progression in July 2020, she began Xeloda until February 2021, when she was taken off of it, primarily because of hand/foot syndrome and disease progression. She then began Faslodex and Piqray but had trouble tolerating Piqray by March 2021.

As of April 2021, Judith and her oncologist were working to make this combination more tolerable. If she cannot tolerate the treatment or if it does induce remission, a new treatment regimen will be recommended. Genetic sequencing from a liquid (blood) biopsy found a BRCA mutation shed into the blood from the tumor. This might allow for an attempt at treatment with one of the PARP inhibitors, another alternative to IV cytoxic therapy.

To date, Judith has had MBC for eleven years. Her only chemotherapy to date is the oral drug Xeloda.

5, Judith: Takeaway

Judith has lived eleven years with MBC and has received eight different forms of treatment, with only one of those being chemotherapy (Xeloda). This form of chemotherapy is orally administered. At this juncture, however, if her current treatment with Piqray and Faslodex does not control her disease, it may be time to move on to intravenous chemotherapy. Many drugs are available including Taxol (or Abraxane), Gemzar, Eribulin, Navelbine, Doxil (or low-dose weekly Adriamycin), Taxotere, and Ixempra. Thus, even after eleven years of treatment for MBC, Judith still has many more options available to induce remission and prolong life.

Even now, as we start to contemplate intravenous chemotherapy, next-generation sequencing *may* have provided another non-chemotherapy oral option. Using a so-called liquid biopsy (blood test), it appears her cancer is shedding a mutated BRCA gene into the bloodstream. These tumor-related genes are called somatic mutations. Of note, after discovering this mutation, her oncologist performed classical genetic testing and did *not* find this mutation. Thus, this is a somatic mutation found only in the tumor but not in every cell in the body (genetic). However, there are data suggesting that somatic mutations may respond to PARP inhibitors (olaparib and talazoparib) (28).

My Cancer Journey: Judith's Story

Most people would likely have to try hard to imagine the shock of receiving a cancer diagnosis. It would probably be beyond their imagination to think about a stage 4 diagnosis.

I was first diagnosed with breast cancer in February of 2001. I found the lump in my breast on February 1, my twin boys' twelfth birthday. A day that was previously filled with the wonderment of their miracle conception and premature birth was temporarily changed into a day of intense fear and sadness for me.

I knew immediately that my life from that moment on was forever changed. What I did not know was that there would be many years of blessings and gifts beyond my wildest dreams waiting for me.

About five years after chemotherapy, and after twenty-five years of marriage, my husband and I decided to divorce.

I was in search of who Judith was now. In light of my cancer history, who was this woman, mother, and daughter? I began to build a life on my own that I had never lived. It was actually scary—not as scary as cancer, but scary. I had no medical insurance and stopped taking tamoxifen.

This was a bad decision, balanced by suddenly feeling like a new woman, physically and emotionally. However, I do not recommend this. Do not go off the medication. Discuss with your doctor and follow their recommendations.

Fast-forward to the spring of 2010, I began to notice very tiny bumps on my right breast. I thought they were bites of some sort. The bites seemed to grow in size. Finally, I saw a dermatologist a week before my birthday in October of 2010. She performed a biopsy. On my birthday one week later, I was notified that the result was cancer. I was fifty-eight years old.

I went into a tailspin and totally broke down. I thought about planning my funeral—what should I wear? Who will I invite? Do I throw a big party? Where's the cancer manual when ya need it?!

My sons, who were twenty-one by this time, brought me back to reality. My incredible sons lifted me up and reminded me that I was strong! They were incredibly strong too! They joined the fight yet again, and they continue to be my partners on this journey.

I found an oncologist near me, but after a month, I decided to go to UM Sylvester for a second opinion.

I met with Dr. Vogel in January of 2011, and he went into detail about the treatment plan ahead and how a diagnosis of stage 4 cancer would affect me. I asked brutal questions, and he gave me answers. I was so emotionally frazzled that I totally forgot most of the answers! The survival numbers were in small numbers, not thousands. Hearing those numbers, my fear began to lessen.

What I recall was that I was filled with hope. This hope allowed me to find strength again.

I did go off another medication after a long period of success due to severe tailbone pain. Don't do that either. While the pain disappeared, the cancer didn't.

Somehow, though, I'm still here, and to me, that is unbelievable. It is a testament to all the breakthroughs with modern medicine, coupled with a will to live my life. Possibly, we can consider metastatic breast cancer as we do other chronic diseases; it can be managed with appropriate medications, and we can continue to live.

So what has kept me going these last ten-plus years with stage 4 disease?

First and foremost—prayer! My parents named me after St. Jude, patron saint of hopeless cases and things despaired of. Pretty accurate; however, hopeless is not the state of mind or heart that I would ever choose to be in! But my prayers have been answered!

Back in 2001, during chemo, I prayed that I would live to see my sons through high school. They had just started middle school when I was diagnosed. I knew they needed me, and I needed to help them find their way in the world. That's all I wanted. That prayer has been answered as well.

One day back in the summer of 2001, I was feeling very sorry for myself. The chemotherapy was affecting my eyes, and I was lying on the couch wanting a normal life again. I went to open the blinds even though I knew it would hurt my eyes. On the window was an angel sun catcher that my brother Christopher had given me when I first was diagnosed. I looked at that sun catcher. In that very instant, I felt at peace, and I realized a very important truth.

What was the point of the experience if there wasn't something important to discover on the journey?

Why go through the process if there wasn't something amazing waiting on the other side of treatment?

Was the point of cancer just suffering or trudging through the muck?

No, that just couldn't be the point of it all. I knew there was something that was going to come to me, and I began building my faith in my journey.

These years of treatment have provided me with insights, soul growth, laughter, joy, and blessings.

My twin sons, Billy and Danny, are my rocks when I need someone to tie my line to. They keep me from going too far out. They've scolded me, loved me, and cracked jokes. Their humor can bring about those wonderful belly laughs. They take me to my treatments, check on me throughout the day, and I always feel their love.

My ex-husband went through my first cancer experience with me and has kept our family going with his strength and steady optimism. He has taken me to many of my appointments. God bless him!

Another thing that has helped me as I make my way through this incredible journey, and I can't stress this enough, is a sense of humor. While many may not find dealing with cancer funny, and I don't always view it as comical; there are many times that cancer is funny for me. If I can joke about it, so can others, and they can see and share in my journey on my terms.

My terms. One of the best gifts of this journey—I do this on my terms. It's my body, my mind, and my soul that fights this battle, and that is incredibly empowering. Cancer is a struggle for our souls—it can be a lonely one-on-one fight at times. When all is said and done, I will not let cancer reduce my power, define who I am, or lessen the strength of my spirit.

If you are struggling with the diagnosis, please know in your heart and soul that we *are* with you.

So many of us are sharing this journey together! You are not alone, and so many of us are with you!

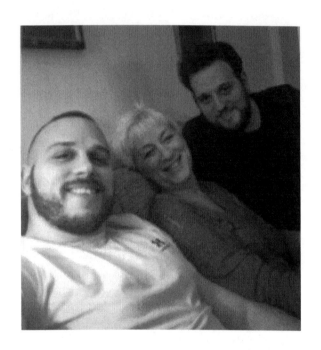

6: Mildred

In July 2005, at age seventy, Mildred was diagnosed with infiltrating ductal carcinoma of the right breast. It was 1.7 cm, ER positive and PR positive, and HER2 negative. Ultimately, a mastectomy was necessary as the margins at the time of the lumpectomy were involved. She did not desire reconstruction.

Mildred received adjuvant tamoxifen from March 2006 to January 2010 and stopped when she was diagnosed with a solitary bone metastasis. Biopsy of the right iliac bone showed disease that was ER positive and PR positive. Due to discomfort in the hip, she received radiation therapy for pain relief and then tamoxifen withdrawal (27). This lasted from January 2010 to April 2011 when she was found to have progression in bone. In 2010, she also started on Xgeva, last given in July 2014. It should be noted that Mildred's tamoxifen withdrawal of seventeen months was the longest I have seen. She could be considered stage 4 NED (see chapter 3), as her only site of disease was radiated when she began tamoxifen withdrawal.

In April 2011, she began therapy with anastrozole and remained on that for the next eight years until she developed new bone lesions in the sternum and skull. Mildred was asymptomatic, and thus anastrozole was continued until the skull lesion enlarged further on imaging. In April 2019, brain MRI indicated that the right parietal skull lesion had associated thickening of the meninges beneath the bone, and radiation was delivered to the area, completed in May 2019.

In July 2019, a repeat MRI showed the possibility of a new metastasis in another bone of the skull base, and this is being followed closely.

Fulvestrant and Ibrance were begun in August 2021 and continue as of March 2021.

Thus, Mildred has had MBC for eleven years and has not required chemotherapy at all with an initial diagnosis of breast cancer sixteen years prior.

6, Mildred: Takeaway

At first relapse, the initial treatment was simply stopping tamoxifen (e.g., tamoxifen withdrawal). This interesting phenomenon was also discussed in chapter 3 and chapter 5, referenced previously in a publication by Howell et al. (27). The withdrawal response lasted 17 months after stopping tamoxifen in January 2020. Her next therapeutic maneuver, anastrozole, controlled her disease for eight years and three months. As of December 2020, Mildred has had metastatic disease for almost eleven years and has yet to require chemotherapy.

Mildred's Story

I was diagnosed with breast cancer fourteen years ago and underwent a mastectomy. With help and guidance, I was in remission for eight years. When I developed cancer in my iliac bone, I received five days of radiation. After cancer was discovered in the skull and was painful, I again was treated with radiation.

I am being treated with new medications. I have received shots and pills that keep me going.

Support and encouragement is what one needs for one's journey. We should believe in the power of positive thinking, as it is a new ball game each day.

Cancer cannot take our life, and we must try to keep ourselves occupied. That is the key to survival.

Friends and family and my medical team have been helping me in my journey and recovery. I will beat the disease.

Every day is a new beginning with faith, hope, and sunshine in our heart.

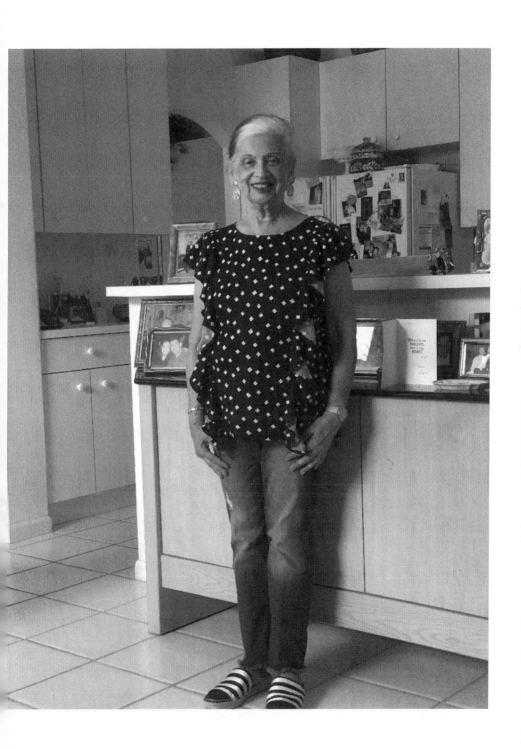

7: Joanne

In 1998, at age thirty-eight, Joanne underwent bilateral mastectomies and reconstruction for invasive breast cancer.

Two years later, in 2000, she developed a recurrence in the bone and was treated in North Florida from 2000 to December 2004. Sequentially, she received low-dose Adriamycin and anastrozole, Lupron and Faslodex, and then Aromasin.

In 2004, she received radiation to the base of her skull for metastatic disease with pain.

Subsequently, in early 2005, Joanne was diagnosed with a positive lymph node in her neck. Additional imaging noted cancer in the sternum that responded well to a combination of Taxotere and Xeloda.

Joanne's doctors gave her a chemotherapy holiday with good control on tamoxifen from April 2005 to November 2005. She then underwent radiation therapy to the sternum.

At this time, she transferred her care to our service. She restarted Xeloda from December 2005 to July 2006, with Navelbine added in July 2006 due to increased activity in the right chest wall. The combination of Navelbine and Xeloda was stopped in July 2006 for a drug holiday, while she was in remission.

Estradiol was started in December 2006, but letrozole was substituted in August 2007.

In 2009, due to progression on imaging, surgical excision of the anterior third rib was performed, as this was the only area of active tumor. It was ER+/PR–. Letrozole was continued as she had no evidence of disease progression elsewhere in the body, and the residual disease had been excised.

Imaging indicated supraclavicular nodal involvement in September 2009. Tamoxifen was given until July 2010 when, again, progression was noted.

Tamoxifen withdrawal was instituted until further progression in March 2011.

Monthly Faslodex was begun, and letrozole was added in July 2011 when she developed a new lesion while continuing Faslodex.

Although Joanne had received Xgeva because of bone metastasis, she ultimately developed osteonecrosis of the jaw, and so therapy was discontinued.

Joann continues in remission on Faslodex plus letrozole as of June 2021.

She was diagnosed with MBC over sixteen years ago and has been on Faslodex and letrozole for the past nine years, living a normal life.

7, Joanne: Takeaway

For the first five years of treatment for MBC, Joanne was under the care of others. During that time, perhaps her disease was behaving a bit more aggressively as the doctors seemed to place more reliance on chemotherapy regimens including Adriamycin and Taxotere plus Xeloda. In general, the main treatment for ER positive PR negative HER2 negative disease is hormonal with chemotherapy reserved for visceral crisis. This is typically defined as extensive and rapid progression of liver or lung metastases or in patients with such widespread debilitating bone metastases that aggressive chemotherapy is warranted up front. Perhaps Joanne's bone metastases were much worse in 2000, needing more aggressive treatments. Regardless, her fifteen-year battle with MBC has been highlighted by a nine-year period of disease control on the combination of fulvestrant (Faslodex) and letrozole (Femara), indicating just how sensitive her cancer is to hormonal therapy.

Joanne's Story

There will come a day when you will not think about cancer every moment of your day.

I appreciate the many caring and helpful nurses who helped me through my cancer journey.

My breast cancer was a shock to me. I was healthy and young. As my brother said when I was diagnosed with cancer, "For you to get cancer ..."—a person who had a healthy lifestyle and a clean diet, no smoking, drinking, or drugs. Everyone is vulnerable to this disease. So you push on and learn how to navigate through the health care system. Find doctors who specialize in your disease. It is an education. Early on, I learned the importance of finding doctors you have confidence in, you are able to communicate with, and who have your best interest at hand. There are many ups and downs to cancer.

You learn about yourself and how kindness to yourself and others is healing. I find gratitude and joy in every day. In closing, to Dr. Vogel, who has said to me that patients give doctors too much credit. I respectfully disagree. Thank you.

8: Georjean

Georjean was forty-seven years old in November 2000 and had received most of her initial breast cancer treatment at Dartmouth University. She had a left breast tumor, 8 mm in size with negative nodes. It was an invasive ductal carcinoma, ER positive PR positive HER2 negative. Radiation therapy was completed, but she refused chemotherapy and hormonal therapy for this small lesion.

In March 2006, she was diagnosed with another left breast mass that was an infiltrating ductal carcinoma with biopsy-proven bone metastasis in the sixth thoracic vertebrae. Other bony sites were also noted.

Georjean was enrolled in a clinical trial of a novel taxane, Tocosol, and she received that drug from April 2006 to October 2006 at which time she had disease progression.

Following the trial, she was placed on letrozole with Zoladex to suppress ovarian function. After becoming postmenopausal, she continued on letrozole alone until the present time with no evidence of progressive disease, now fourteen years later.

Zometa was given for several years but tolerated poorly. She tried another agent, Xgeva, but also could not tolerate this either and thus is receiving no bone-healing agents.

In 2016, ten years later after diagnosis of MBC with a large left breast mass and bone metastases, Georjean moved to Florida and continued on letrozole.

In May 2017, a bone scan revealed only a skull lesion, which correlated with a 2.8 cm lytic lesion on x-ray. PET scan has been used to follow her radiographically. The breast mass measured only 1.6 cm on imaging while on physical exam, it measures closer to 6 cm. It has been stable since she moved to Florida. While there are lesions in the liver, some are cysts, and some are too small to better characterize. All have been stable over the years. At the sixth thoracic vertebrae, she has a mixed sclerotic and lytic lesion measuring 1.1X1.2 cm.

In spite of the findings of the breast mass on physical examination and stable bone metastasis, as of March 2021, Georjean remains in remission on letrozole for about 15 years. She seems to be living in symbiosis with her large breast mass.

8, Georjean: Takeaway

When your doctor cites statistics, one is that the average duration of control of MBC with aromatase inhibitors is within the fourteen- to sixteen-month range. *However*, no patient is a statistic, and this chapter should clearly point out that any patient with MBC can defy the statistics of disease control. So far in this chapter, we have Georgjean, controlled for 15 years; Joanne, for nine; Mildred, for eight; and Patrice, for eleven years on a given hormonal manipulation.

Take heart, although the survival statistics in MBC may be lower than desired, *you are not a statistic.*

Georjean's Twenty-Year Journey with Breast Cancer

I celebrated the start of the year 2000 filled with joy and hope for the new century. However, during a yearly checkup in October, my primary care physician palpated a small lump in my left breast. A needle biopsy confirmed that it was cancer. As I was forty-five years old at the time, I decided to undergo a lumpectomy followed by radiation. I went back to work within days. I was a marketing director at the time for a computer company and traveled to Europe once a month for years. I was cured and had five years of normal mammograms and checkups.

Unfortunately, my mammogram six years later after diagnosis indicated microcalcifications. Numerous tests revealed that I had a large tumor in my left breast, as well as a tumor in my spine and one at my skull. It was the same type of breast cancer as my initial diagnosis, estrogen positive and HER2 negative.

I was heartbroken when I was diagnosed with stage IV breast cancer. Why me? No one in my family had ever experienced breast cancer. I felt great, ate a healthy diet, and exercised. After discussing treatment options with my doctor, I chose to fight my cancer with chemotherapy. I changed the ringtone on my phone to the song "Staying Alive." My husband was my biggest supporter. He took me every week for my treatments and stayed with me during my chemotherapy sessions, which lasted for six months.

The statistics that I found on the internet for survival were pretty scary. I decided to keep a positive attitude! My brothers included me in prayer circles at their churches as I progressed through my treatments. I tried a visualization technique during each weekly chemo session. I pictured tiny soldiers surrounding and fighting each cancer cell. My checkup scans eventually showed that the tumor in my breast was gone, that my bone tumors were stable, and that there was no disease progression. As I finished six months of chemotherapy, a new breast MRI showed what was believed to be a new tumor. My doctor ordered a biopsy immediately. I couldn't believe that this was happening, after all the good results. I was prepped for the procedure and was lying there waiting. The doctor who was to perform the biopsy came in asked me to go to another room for an ultrasound first. While I was waiting for the doctor, I said a prayer. He came in and couldn't find anything suspicious on the ultrasound! Everything looked fine. He told me that I could go home. I no longer needed any more chemotherapy treatments and went on a maintenance course of treatment.

My husband and I splurged and went to Hawaii for Valentine's Day after I was finished with chemo. My doctors kept telling me that the cancer would outsmart the Femara that I am taking daily and that my cancer would return. I traveled and visited my family and friends whenever I could, thinking that it could be the last time that I would see them.

I still take a Femara tablet every day. I had quarterly Zometa infusions for seven years, which were replaced by Xgeva injections for two years. I stopped getting the injections three years ago, due to side effects.

I had an amazing team of doctors and nurses for seventeen years at Dartmouth Medical Center and Foundation Medical Partners in New Hampshire. We decided to retire and move to Florida at the end of 2016. My oncologist recommended the wonderful team at the Sylvester Cancer Center.

Having cancer changed my life. I am grateful for each day, and I no longer get upset or annoyed by trivial things. I laugh when I see others laugh. I try to show kindness to everyone. I lost my husband and best friend a few months ago to a heart attack.

It has been fourteen years now, and my checkups have all been fine; the cancer has not returned. I am still keeping a positive attitude. I guess that I should change the ringtone on my phone to "I'm Still Standing" now.

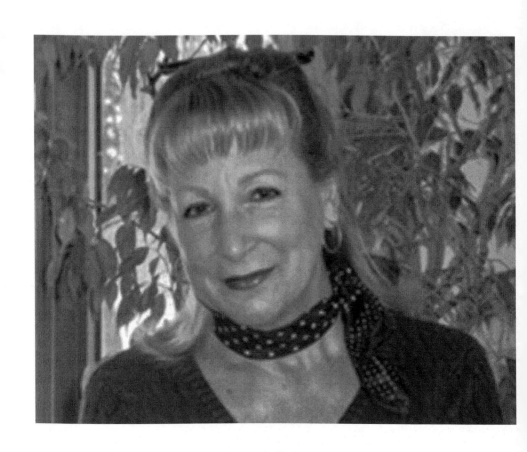

9: Linda

At age sixty-one, Linda underwent chemotherapy for a large tumor in the left breast. She was treated with Adriamycin and Cytoxan followed by Taxol. She then underwent a left breast modified mastectomy followed by radiation and five years of exemestane (Aromasin).

In September 2011, she was found to have metastatic disease to the bone and received Faslodex and Xgeva for over five years until disease progression in December 2016.

Letrozole was started in December 2016, and Ibrance was added in January 2017. Although she experienced a femur fracture in July 2018, she remained on therapy.

As of December 2020, Linda has lived with MBC for nine years and has not required chemotherapy.

9, Linda: Takeaway

Linda was on first line fulvestrant hormonal therapy for over five years for MBC. Although not included in this compilation of patients, another woman, Lorraine, not included in this book, had disease control on fulvestrant for eight years. Thus, while statistics would predict for disease control on a given hormonal manipulation for less than two years, in the cases of Linda and Lorraine, disease control on fulvestrant lasted for five and eight years, respectively.

In addition, Linda has achieved continued response on second line hormonal therapy with letrozole and Ibrance. Although with MBC for nine years to date, she has not yet received chemotherapy for her MBC.

10: Catherine

In 1991, at age thirty-three, Catherine underwent a right lumpectomy for an 8 cm tumor with nine positive lymph nodes. The tumor was ER and PR positive and HER2 negative.

She received Adriamycin-based chemotherapy followed by high-dose chemotherapy as well as a bone marrow transplant at a cancer center. This was followed by radiation and, ultimately, tamoxifen for five years.

Of note, she has a history of papillary thyroid carcinoma treated with resection followed by radioactive iodine therapy. This has been in remission since 2003. This was not long after the diagnosis of Hodgkin's lymphoma in her daughter, Katchen, in 2000. At this time, it appears Katchen has been cured.

At the time of diagnosis of microinvasive cervical carcinoma in 1992, Catherine underwent a total hysterectomy and removal of the ovaries and has had no further issues.

Regarding the breast cancer, in 2005 (fourteen years after her initial diagnosis), she developed metastatic disease to the right lower lobe of the lung with associated lymph node involvement. Catherine experienced disease control from 2005 to 2013 on letrozole. Unfortunately, during these years, she lost her mother and father to cancer in 2008 and 2010.

Unfortunately, Catherine progressed in 2013 and she took fulvestrant from July 2013 to 2017. From 2014 to 2016, while coping with her own medical issues, she had other struggles. She was a caregiver for her significant other who ultimately succumbed to a very rare tumor.

In June 2017, she underwent a biopsy of the right lower lobe nodule. The pathology confirmed metastatic breast carcinoma consistent with a breast primary. It was ER positive, PR positive, and HER2 negative.

As Catherine lives far from the clinic, she is seen infrequently. In 2017, at the time of the lung recurrence Kisqali and letrozole was proposed, but she declined. She accepted tamoxifen rechallenge instead. Surgical resection was also considered for the right lower lung mass, but she declined to proceed

During 2018, Catherine stopped tamoxifen and began vitamins and naturopathic therapy.

In 2019, she was diagnosed with liver metastasis and a biopsy once again confirmed that the cells were ER positive, PR negative and HER2 negative.

In May 2019, she started Navelbine and Xeloda. She also continued on naturopathic therapy, which involved IV vitamin C among other treatments. She has a very close relationship with her naturopath provider.

Catherine continued the combination of Navelbine and Xeloda for six months, though she experienced hand/foot syndrome, which led to reductions of Xeloda dosing. In October 2019, disease progression was suspected, and she was switched to letrozole and Ibrance. Due to increased symptoms of lower back pain and cough, she discontinued these drugs in November 2019. She returned to Navelbine and Xeloda in November of 2019. However, by December 2019, she had significant disease progression in the liver and began Gemzar and Taxol. After two days, Catherine was hospitalized. She required therapeutic and palliative paracentesis to draw fluid from her distended abdomen. Of note, cancer was not discovered in the fluid.

She elected to discontinue naturopathic medicine at that time.

After Gemzar and Taxol, over several months in 2020, she received Abraxane with intolerable side effects and fulvestrant and Verzenio with intolerable side effects even at a low dose. After one dose of Talzenna, she experienced extreme nausea, difficulty walking, and somnolence. While visiting her daughter, Jessie, in Oregon, she sought opinions from oncologists in Oregon. This team recommended a Talzenna dose reduction, and then when scans showed further progression, they recommended Taxol.

After just a few weeks of Taxol, on October 27, 2020, Catherine passed away just weeks before the birth of her first grandchild. Catherine lived with MBC for fifteen years.

10, Catherine: Takeaway

Catherine has always been an independent thinker. She was treated for three different cancers, including cervical cancer, thyroid cancer, and breast cancer. Interestingly, several of her roommates in college also developed cancer of various types at similar ages. Catherine investigated this troubling cluster of cancer among young women, but it is unclear if there was any connection.

Her own story of MBC has been a remarkable one, a fifteen-plus years journey. During the first eight years, Catherine took hormonal therapy. Her three years on fulvestrant also exceeded the average.

After twelve years of control on hormonal therapy, the last three years were more difficult. Struggling with both metastatic cancer and an infection in the lung, illnesses in multiple family members, and the additional responsibilities of caring for her significant other took a toll on Catherine.

While relying heavily on a mix of conventional and naturopathic medicines, she finally abandoned naturopathic therapy in December 2019.

More recently, blood samples were evaluated and revealed BRCA1 mutations. Of course, because of Catherine's age and family history, she had genomic testing for BRCA and was found to be negative. However, these next-generation tests identify *somatic* mutations. Thus, while her cancer is expressing BRCA1 mutation, the remainder of the cells in her body (genomic mutations) do not.

We now have drugs, PARP inhibitors, which are approved to treat genomic mutation carriers with MBC. There are data indicating that BRCA somatic mutations might also be susceptible to these drugs. Indeed, a recently published metanalysis indicated that the response rate to PARP inhibitors for germline carriers was 69/157 (43.9%) *but* was also 24/43 (55.8%) for somatic carriers (30).

In September 2020, a PET scan showed reasonable control with Faslodex and Verzenio. Unfortunately, she was found to have intolerable Verzenio toxicity. It was recommended to add the PARP inhibitor Talzenna to fulvestrant. Unfortunately, by the time she decided to start this regimen, she left to visit her daughter in Oregon. While in Oregon, the pace of her disease accelerated, ultimately robbing the world of this young and vibrant woman, who could best be described as a delightful, free-thinking force of nature.

Catherine's Story

I was diagnosed at thirty-two years old with stage 2, estrogen receptor positive breast cancer. There was an 8 cm lump in my right breast, large enough that I discovered it myself. There were also nine lymph nodes under my arm that were noted to contain cancer. I was "healthy as a horse," my mother kept saying, a strong young mother of two with no family history. Through the process of diagnosis, each doctor expressed their surprise. In 1990, I was considered to be too young to have breast cancer. I underwent two surgical procedures. As the grim news was rolling in, I feared death for about a minute, as young people may, then I put it out of my head—I was going to live! My daughters were five and seven, the national statistics for breast cancer had just moved to one in nine women. My daughter Katchen had twenty-seven students in her school class and three of the parents were diagnosed that year! Unfortunately, the other parents did not survive. I saw a luminary Friday night memorializing one of them on the track. My doctors recommended the most aggressive treatment at the time, which was six rounds of chemo followed by bone marrow rescue, and then six weeks of radiation, concluding with five years of tamoxifen.

The following year, I was diagnosed with cervical cancer, and because of the nature of the breast cancer, it was recommended that I have a hysterectomy and removal of my ovaries. I still miss them. Even though it may have been a blessing, I was considered in remission and cancer-free! Twelve years later, I was diagnosed with thyroid cancer, possibly fallout from radiation.

During follow-up for the thyroid cancer, metastatic breast cells were found in the mediastinal nodes of my chest. I went on a drug called Femara, an estrogen inhibitor. I had clean scans a few months later and then years of relief until spring of 2017 when I started wheezing and having shortness of breath.

Spread of cancer to the lungs was the diagnosis this time. The surgeon recommended that I have two lobes of my right lung removed. Thank God he had to go to Prague and couldn't do that right away.

So, if you are keeping count, now we are at five! All really from the original diagnosis!

So, this is not what I wanted to talk about, but I felt the need to give you a little background. There is so much more.

From the very first diagnosis, I was determined to take charge of my treatment. I will always remember a powerful thing that a friend said to me: "This is your cancer, not your doctor's, not your mother's or father's, not your husband's—it is yours."

Sure, I went through the "why me?" I'm blaming myself for where I have lived or what I have eaten. The nutritionist in the oncologist office put me on a special diet. I gained thirty pounds in a few years' time.

I had a relatively healthy, crunchy, whole-wheat diet before that and thought there must be more. I tried macrobiotics and vegan, read everything, and soon went back to life and left mainstream.

After the diagnosis of thyroid cancer, I started seeing a naturopathic provider in New Hampshire. The diet and treatments were for my blood type and cleansing and detoxifying. I took an arsenal of vitamins for years, and although it kept the tumor at bay, I wasn't successful in eradicating it, so I chose to have surgery two years later. For years I have stayed with the premise of the diet, but slowly and surely slipped back into some relaxed habits!

I also feel that my belief in a higher power and my practice of a spiritual path started from the first diagnosis. I read books on visualization and used scrubbing bubbles during chemo to see my body being cleaned out of cancer. I started to use music and meditation to calm me during my five weeks in isolation in the bone marrow unit, and I believed strongly in my body's ability to overcome this disease, even though it seemed that I was one of those blow-up clowns that you could punch over but they would always stand back up!

The best way for me to take my power back was to control my prognosis! The doctors can give you a diagnosis, but the prognosis was mine.

At one point, I read Myrtle Fillmore's *Healing Letters* and Emily Cady's *Lessons in Truth*, and the resonating theme for me was that this disease was not my truth! Cancer is not the truth about me! I am a powerful healing child of God, and I radiate perfect health!

Back to the past year, having outlived two doctors in Key West, I went back to my original oncologist (I had to do a lot of forgiveness work with him as he said some very stupid things to me through the years, including not telling me about diminishing scan results), "You can run, but you can't hide" top in the field of breast cancer! I realize that he only sees a sick woman. Dr. Vogel did not recommend lung surgery, switched my hormone to in end-stage drug called Faslodex, monthly injections that block estrogen and have numerous side effects that I will get to a little later. In general, they do this until it doesn't work and more. It all sounded pretty grim. I also went back to the naturopathic provider in New Hampshire. He had a much brighter outlook.

The provider I saw, had branched out on his own and was specializing in cancer. He recommended a ketogenic diet completely sugar-free, high fat, and all organic. In his words, "beating cancer is a full-time job." I also was prescribed a regimen of herbs and supplements to support the immune system and kill cancer cells around thirty pills a meal.

I started both the diet and supplements and the injections in July of this year. Oddly enough, the oncologist agreed with the ketogenic diet approach, and for the first time, I also saw an integrative oncologist. What a blessing that there is someone integrating the fields of mind body and cancer! I was able to take him my protocol from the naturopathic and get his opinion. In the past, there was no reconciling these two worlds.

The naturopathic provider, however, was not a fan of the Faslodex, so this decision to do both was mine—they all are—and I think it is important to note that even when I have tried to heal myself with natural treatments, I have had scans and doctors who followed me here in Key West, never dismissed any treatment I was doing; other doctors I have encountered have been a little more fear-filled!)

The studies done on the ketogenic diet included hyperbaric oxygen treatment, so I bought my own chamber and spent an hour a day in the chamber.

The premise is that the cells in the body become hyper-oxygenated, and cancer cells cannot thrive in an oxygen-rich environment. It is very relaxing, and I use the time to rest and meditate.

I continued my yoga practice and teaching. Yoga has always been a part of my life, and the practice centers me and allows me to find inner strength and courage during treatment.

I continued singing as much as possible, chanting the many names of God with Krishna Das, Deva Premal, and Snatam Kaur, playing our positive music in my home and singing in church. I even attended the unity music conference.

I had acupuncture every other week to bring my energy and immunity up and massage from my sister-in-law every week to stimulate my immune system. I had Reiki treatments here at church, and I remembered to tap when any fear started to creep in. And there was fear! For the first time ever, I thought I may not make it through this time, but I assembled my team of practitioners to support me, and I was not alone.

I rested, I prayed, I shopped, and I cooked! I isolated a bit and hunkered down for the battle. I sent my menu out to friends and family. I told people I needed their support.

Beating cancer is a full-time job.

Because I started both programs simultaneously, I was never quite sure what was causing the side effects. The internet, both a blessing and a curse, brought me way too much information on the Faslodex side effects and statistics. I had joint pain and muscle fatigue and severe stomach issues, and I attributed them to the drug, but then eventually had to take a break from the supplements to correct my stomach. I was the only one who was truly integrating here! My body was the experiment.

The first scans in October showed signs of shrinking and diminishing tumors in my lungs! I was happy but a bit discouraged and kept up with the program. The PET in December showed no signs of cancer!

I believe in an integrative approach, and because that is my belief as we teach here, that is what will work for me!

I believe that we are whole and individual women, and we need to be treated that way

I believe in a power and a source greater than me that knows my wholeness.

I believe that diet and nutrition, rest and inner work are key to healing through cancer, and these are all things that one can do proactively to keep oneself healthy.

It helps me to take my power back away from this disease and to see myself through it.

Finding doctors that you can resonate with and who are open to the mystery.

I find, in writing all this down, a deep sense of gratitude to my family. I am blessed with the ability to afford healthcare and the ridiculous out-of-pocket expenses that go along with a diagnosis such as this. There were challenges getting the bone marrow transplant approved by insurance. I have had the same insurance until Affordable Care Act allowed me to switch to a better plan. My expenses for the naturopathic and the supplements are not covered. Our business allowed me to not work for several months and truly focus on healing, family members picking up the slack. I felt supported by friends here at church and afar in prayer.

Evelyn and the prayer team worked overtime to lift me up. Melody supported me in singing my truth here at church.

Thank you all for listening. I have never flown the banner of survivor because I feel that we all have our own path.

This was mine.

I hope it will be helpful to some to see my strength, hope, and courage!

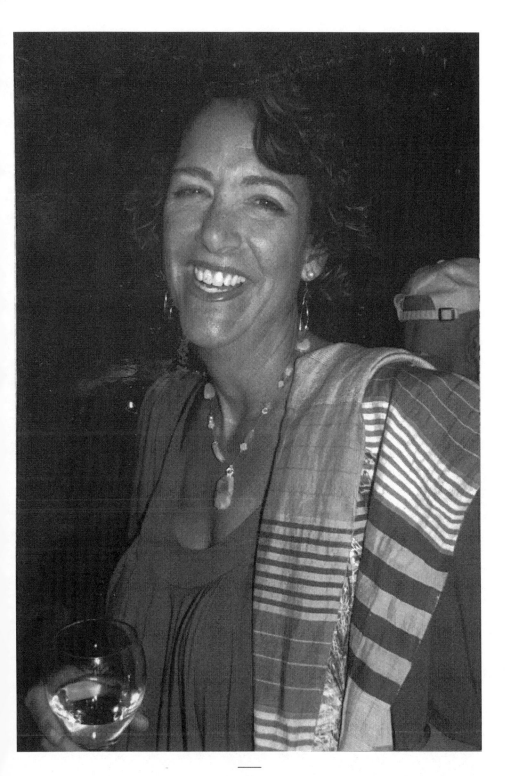

CHAPTER VI

HER2-Positive Breast Cancer

Introduction

The 1990s were years of great anticipation after the discovery by Dr. Dennis Slamon that HER2 can become a cancer-causing gene. We all have HER2 in every cell in our body. We inherit one copy from each parent. Like every gene in our body, HER2 has a normal function. However, approximately 15% of breast cancers have cells that, instead of carrying two copies of HER2, have been amplified and carry many more copies of the gene, converting the good gene into an oncogene. The pharmaceutical company Genentech (collaborating with Dr. Slamon) synthesized the compound trastuzumab (Herceptin). This drug has revolutionized the treatment of HER2-amplified (+) breast cancer. When first discovered, HER2 positive breast cancer was one of the more virulent forms of the disease. Over the past twenty-five years, additional HER2 drugs have been developed. Now, HER2 positive disease has a better prognosis. HER2 positive MBC patients can have disease control for a decade or longer. These women can be conundrums for doctors and patients alike. Dare we think, perhaps, that we could discontinue their anti-HER2 therapy and consider the word *cure* regarding HER2 positive MBC? In my practice, there are several such patients, and each year, the question is raised: Stop or continue? Some have stopped and remain disease-free (dare we hope cured). More frequently, patients are ingrained with the thought that MBC is incurable and elect to continue maintenance indefinitely. You will meet these women in this and other chapters, including Gloria in chapter 4.

Currently, triple-positive MBC disease has been found to have a better prognosis than other breast cancer subtypes, except for luminal A (31). We are able to target both the estrogen receptor and the HER2 pathways, and thus there are a large number of therapeutic options. The addition of cytotoxic chemotherapy further expands choices for this group.

Early stage HER2 positive breast cancer patients who are also hormone-receptor negative are more likely to achieve complete disappearance of the cancer (63.2% vs. 27.3%) when given chemotherapy with targeted therapy prior to surgery than patients with triple-positive disease (32).

1: Anne-Marie

Anne-Marie was diagnosed at age thirty-nine in 2001 with HER2 positive primary breast cancer. She was treated on a clinical trial with Adriamycin and Cytoxan followed by Taxotere and Herceptin or a placebo. She underwent lumpectomy and radiation as well.

She then received adjuvant tamoxifen from 2001 to 2004 and switched to anastrozole from 2004 to 2010. She developed metastatic disease to bone in 2010, treated initially with lapatinib (Tykerb), exemestane, and Xeloda from March 2010 to October 2010 when there was progression in the spine.

Anne-Marie received Herceptin and Tykerb from October 2010 to May 2014. While in remission, Tykerb was discontinued, and she was maintained on Herceptin alone until progression at L5.

Tykerb was restarted December 2015, and stereotactic radiosurgery was delivered to the L5 vertebrae.

In April 2017, there was worsening again at L5, and further stereotactic surgery was prescribed as well as kyphoplasty. Kyphoplasty is a procedure performed typically by radiology. A needle is placed into the collapsed vertebra. A balloon is placed and expands the vertebra. Ultimately, cement is put in over the balloon to reconstruct the vertebrae. Systemic therapy was not changed.

Anne-Marie did well for a year. However, in April 2018, a mass was found near her stomach. For the first time, Anne-Marie was feeling ill. She lost her appetite and lost weight. She began Kadcyla, which was discontinued in July 2019 when imaging revealed progression in that area. She experienced nausea, acid reflux, and continued weight loss.

In July 2019, she started Navelbine, Herceptin, and Perjeta, and immediately she felt dramatically better. Her CEA, a tumor marker that had been her dominant marker, went from 8.3 to 2.4. She gained weight and symptoms resolved. In July 2020, she stopped the Navelbine (a chemo holiday) and continued with Herceptin and Perjeta alone, which continues as of June 2021.

As of June 2021, Anne-Marie has lived with MBC for eleven years and is leading a normal life other than every three-week treatment visits.

1, Anne-Marie: Takeaway

For eleven years, Anne-Marie has experienced good control of her MBC without the need for any drugs which cause hair loss. As a career woman, she travels extensively for business and pleasure. She loves fishing and went fly fishing in Chile two years ago.

Although lapatinib (Tykerb) can at times cause side effects, Anne Marie has had good control for long periods of time with low toxicity.

2: Pat

At age fifty-seven, in 1997, Pat underwent a right mastectomy for stage I, hormone-receptor-positive breast cancer. She received six cycles of CMF in the adjuvant setting, which was completed in August of 1997.

In March 2002, she was diagnosed with metastatic cancer in the liver. She was treated initially with letrozole, but she experienced progression of her disease, prompting a change in therapy to Taxotere and Herceptin. This was given from May to December 2002. Fortunately, this regimen produced a complete response in the liver.

Herceptin continued from December 2002 to the present time without any evidence of recurrent disease.

She is now eighteen years disease-free after only six months of chemotherapy and eighteen years of Herceptin, which continues every three weeks as of June 2021. Pat is another patient possibly cured of her MBC, but with continuing concerns that stopping the drug will lead to cancer recurrence.

2, Pat: Takeaway

Pat is one of the fortunate patients who has experienced prolonged disease control (dare we think cure) of MBC with disease spread to the liver after only six months of chemotherapy and eighteen years of Herceptin every three weeks. We have previously alluded to the conundrum that doctors and patients face as years go by wondering if their disease-free state requires continuation of Herceptin. Of note, one of Dr. Slamon's earliest patients with lung metastasis was treated for about three months with carboplatin, and an uncertain short duration of Herceptin and is disease-free for at least twenty-six years on no antineoplastic therapy.

Pat's Story

My name is Pat Henderson, and I am the mother of four daughters—Tina, Bambi, Kim, and Kelly. My breast cancer journey began in 1997 at the young age of fifty-eight while I was living in Burleson, Texas. At my yearly routine mammogram, I was told that there was a small mass in my left breast. Arrangements were made quickly to have the tumor removed. I started chemotherapy after lumpectomy. After completion of chemo without losing too much hair, I was given a clean bill of health.

Four years later, in 2001, I moved to South Florida to be closer to my daughter Bambi. I saw my oncologist one last time to get my previous records and to say goodbye to my team. While I was there, the oncologist asked if she could do one last breast examination on me. To our surprise, she discovered a small lump, again in the left breast. She removed part of it right there in the office. It was tiny, but nonetheless it was a cancer. I was leaving that afternoon for Florida. I promised that I would find an oncologist as soon as I arrived in Florida.

Once I made it to my new home in Margate, Florida, my daughter Bambi and I saw an oncologist in the practice of Dr. Charles Vogel in Plantation. After evaluation, it was determined that I required a mastectomy. I was treated with radiation and then chemotherapy once again. The radiation was challenging, and I required treatment breaks due to severe skin reaction. I received a total of thirty-six treatments. It was pure hell.

After radiation, I began my chemo sessions. My diagnosis was HER2 positive. I was offered an experimental treatment with chemotherapy and a new drug named Herceptin. I agreed and started treatment right away. This time around, I lost all my beautiful, long black hair by the third treatment. I am now wearing wigs, and I have to say, it's not that bad. I can change my look and hair color daily if I choose to do so.

After three years of Herceptin, I was informed that my insurance would no longer be accepted, and I needed to find another oncologist. I saw Dr. Vogel. He is very compassionate with his patients and always encourages me to keep moving forward with my fight against breast cancer. I eventually started seeing Dr. Mahtani, whom I just adore. She is my hero. I am forever grateful for the care and treatment that I receive from the Sylvester Comprehensive Cancer Center, Deerfield Beach location. I am currently still receiving my Herceptin treatment every three weeks and am hoping to be a candidate for a new injection treatment in the near future. It has been my decision to continue with Herceptin. Every third Wednesday of each month is a fun day when I sit and visit with the nurses and staff and receive my Herceptin. We all tell stories and laugh for two hours. They gave me the nickname of Giggles. They love my British accent!

My daughter Bambi has been with me through this entire cancer process. She joins me for my clinic visits, treatments, and yearly PET scan, which scares me to death. To this day, each PET scan has returned negative, so I will continue to pray for this great news and be positive.

I am eighty-one years old now and consider myself very blessed to still be alive and cancer-free. The Lord is not ready to bring me home yet. I am still living with my daughter Bambi and her husband, Don, in Coconut Creek, Florida.

I am honored that Dr. Vogel and his team had asked me to participate in this book. I'm a twenty-three-year breast cancer survivor, and my life is great. I am happy and healthy.

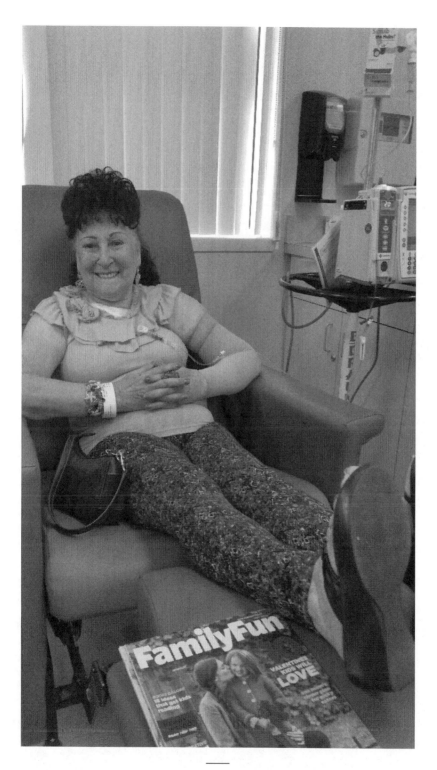

3: Janice

In October 2012 at age seventy, Janice underwent a left breast mastectomy for breast cancer in North Carolina. She did not undergo a workup to look for metastatic cancer prior to her mastectomy. When she returned to her home in Florida, it was discovered that she had disease in her bone and liver. Thus, she had de novo stage 4 disease. It was positive for ER, PR, and HER2.

Herceptin and letrozole were begun in December 2012 and continued to September 2015. Janice had very strong opinions and rejected the concept of cytotoxic chemotherapy at that time.

After three years, she experienced progression. Fulvestrant with Herceptin was given from September 2015 to January 2016. At the next progression, she agreed to chemotherapy. She started on Taxol, Herceptin, and Perjeta, but experienced an allergic reaction to Taxol. She continued on Herceptin and Perjeta alone from January 2013 to May 2018 when a PET scan showed increasing liver lesions, and she had rising tumor markers.

There was only one liver lesion, and it was considered to ablate it and continue Herceptin and Perjeta. Unfortunately, the location of the tumor did not allow for a safe ablation. She began Kadcyla in July 2018. By September 2018, however, at course number 4 after a dose reduction, she noted intolerable side effects, predominantly fatigue. For that reason, she was put back on single agent Herceptin in October 2018. She stayed on Herceptin until the liver lesion grew. She then restarted low dose Kadcyla in June 2019 with a good response.

In September 2019, Janice declined Kadcyla due to feeling ill and insisted on restarting Herceptin. She was maintained on Herceptin until June 2020, when the liver lesion recurred. However, she was still reluctant to change therapies.

As of July 2020, we were bargaining to determine which antitumor treatment she would accept. She declined lapatinib, neratinib, tucatinib, and Xeloda because they are pills. She declined Enhertu because of potential lung toxicity. Thus, as of September 2020, she restarted Kadcyla as she had never progressed on that drug. Again, tumor markers fell, and imaging improved. However, by November, she again requested to be put back on Herceptin. She has been on that drug as of February 2021. By March 2021, markers increased, and imaging confirmed increase in size of her lesions. She once again restarted Kadcyla, again with a decrease in size of her liver lesion.

Janice has lived with MBC for nine years without significant chemotherapy.

3, Janice: Takeaway

Two major publications on trials regarding combined ER and HER2 inhibitors have not been overwhelmingly successful. However, there is no question that some triple positive patients derive benefit from a combination of joint blockade of the HER2 and estrogen receptor pathways (see chapter 6, "Lorraine"). More often than not, this strategy is used in salvage settings. Results from a trial of Taxotere with Herceptin and Perjeta have been impressive in the first line metastatic setting. Thus, doctors are often reluctant to deviate from this care (33). There are, however, patients with multiple comorbidities, advanced age, or strongly stated preferences to avoid cytotoxic chemotherapy for as long as possible that hormonal/HER2 combination options should be covered by third-party payers.

Janice has largely called the shots in her care for the past eight years and has been fortunate to achieve excellent disease control with minimal toxicity. For most, HER2 positive MBC eventually will assume a more aggressive course, and they will ultimately have to choose from effective therapies with some degree of side effects or inconveniences.

4: Lorraine

At age seventy-four in November 2006, Lorraine was diagnosed with infiltrating ductal carcinoma. She underwent a left mastectomy in January 2007 for a 1.7 cm tumor with two positive nodes. Estrogen and progesterone receptors were positive, and HER2 was also positive.

She received anastrozole and Herceptin in the adjuvant setting beginning in February 2007. She completed one year of Herceptin and anastrozole continued until November 2012. It should be mentioned that in 2007, when she took anastrozole with Herceptin, there were no clinical trials to support that course of action. However, her insurance covered the treatment, and she experienced good disease control without the need for chemotherapy.

Interestingly, in April of 2009, Lorraine developed endometrial carcinoma and had removal of her uterus and ovaries for an early-stage uterine cancer. No additional therapy was necessary.

In November 2015, a chest wall mass was noted on physical exam. CT scan was performed and multiple pulmonary nodules were noted suggestive of metastatic disease. There was also involvement of the sternum. After extensive discussions, Lorraine declined treatment. She decided to wait and see the tempo of the disease as she was asymptomatic.

In March 2016, PET scan showed enlargement of the lung nodules, and her CA15-3 increased from 38 to 56. Though she remained asymptomatic, it was felt that therapy was warranted. With no clinical trial supporting data, she was treated in a rather unusual way. Typically, she would start Herceptin at that time. However, she did not want to be tied down to IV medications every three weeks, as she traveled frequently. Around this time, palbociclib was shown to revolutionize the treatment of hormone-receptor positive, HER2 negative disease. Lorraine began letrozole and palbociclib without any anti-HER2 therapy.

As of September 2020, Lorraine had been on letrozole and palbociclib for four years and six months without evidence of recurrent disease and with excellent quality of life.

Unfortunately, routine scans revealed progression in bone. Because of excellent control with hormonal therapy in the past, she started fulvestrant and Herceptin/Hylecta in September 2020, which continues as of June 2021.

Hylecta may be new to the reader. It is a form of Herceptin that can be given via a short infusion under the skin of the thigh. This enabled Lorraine to avoid a port and significantly shortened each visit at the treatment center.

4, Lorraine: Takeaway

Currently, national treatment guidelines and locally designed clinical pathways are ever increasingly guiding our clinical decision-making. Third-party payers adhere to these guidelines. While standardization is optimal, the physician's ability to deviate from these standards of care has become more difficult, and elements of clinical judgement are often superseded by "the rules."

In retrospect, it is unclear how insurance authorization was obtained for adjuvant anastrozole/Herceptin in 2007.However, insurance companies were less stringent at that time.

To date, Lorraine's MBC has taken an indolent course. Tests such as MammaPrint are not approved to aid in decision-making for MBC. However, there are data in early-stage disease that indicate that while classical HER2 testing (IHC and FISH) indicate HER2 positivity, a significant percentage of triple-positive patients studied by MammaPrint actually had luminal intrinsic subtypes and not HER2 (30). These data are certainly hypothesis generating, but study of such patients treated with hormonal therapy alone could be of interest as we speculate which of the two pathways (estrogen receptor or HER2) might predominate in individual patients.

For quality of life, it is appealing to continue to treat with the least toxic therapies possible. So far, Lorraine's quality of life through MBC has been gratifying for her and her physicians.

5: Patricia

In 1996, Patricia, at age fifty-one, presented with stage II node positive breast cancer that was ER positive. HER2 was not available. She received radiation therapy after lumpectomy, which was followed by anastrozole without chemotherapy.

In the year 2000, she relapsed with HER2 positive disease which was treated with Navelbine and Herceptin with dramatic response. This continued until December 2008, when she experienced disease progression. Navelbine was stopped, and Herceptin was continued.

At the next relapse in March 2009, Patricia was switched to Herceptin and Tykerb.

In October 2011, she had progressive disease with new contralateral right breast lesions. These were resected, and she continued on therapy with Tykerb and Herceptin, but Xeloda was added.

Patricia completed six months of Xeloda in April 2012. It was stopped, but Tykerb and Herceptin continued.

As of March 2021, aside from some intermittent variations in Tykerb dosing, she has been in good control of her metastatic disease for eight years. She is now twenty-two years after her initial presentation and twenty years after diagnosis of metastatic disease. It is eight years since her last dose of chemotherapy, which was oral chemotherapy with capecitabine (Xeloda). She has been on Tykerb for almost ten years.

5, Patricia: Takeaway

Patricia has lived with triple-positive MBC for twenty years. She has been maintained solely with anti-HER2 therapy with Tykerb and Herceptin for the past eight years and without chemotherapy for the past twelve years.

With the development of new anti-HER2 drugs such as Perjeta, Kadcyla, neratinib, Enhertu, and tucatinib, Tykerb has been pushed back in our anti-HER2 armamentarium. Burdened with some troublesome side effects, including rash, diarrhea and liver function abnormalities, its dramatic and durable responses are often overlooked. While Herceptin, Perjeta, Kadcyla, and Enhertu target the HER2 receptors on the cell surface and are drugs given by injection, Tykerb, neratinib, and tucatinib interfere with the next step in the HER2 pathway (tyrosine kinase domain) and are pills given by mouth. Blockade with an anti-HER2-receptor drug and a tyrosine kinase inhibitor (TKI; Tykerb) has been shown to be superior to Herceptin alone in a controlled randomized trial in patients with pretreated disease (35). This strategy has proven highly effective for Patricia and many others (including Kelly and Karen in chapter 8 and Anne-Marie in chapter 6). Another advantage of TKIs is their ability to cross the blood-brain barrier and work effectively in brain metastases, a particularly vexing complication of HER2 positive disease. This problem will be discussed further in chapter 8.

6: Marlene

Marlene was initially diagnosed with a well differentiated tubular carcinoma of the left breast in July 1993 at age fifty-three. She underwent a modified mastectomy, showing no residual cancer after the initial biopsy removal and no cancer in her lymph nodes. She underwent an elective prophylactic contralateral mastectomy with reconstructive surgery.

Her cancer was weakly ER positive and had strong progesterone receptors. In 1993, HER2 testing was not performed, but HER2 testing performed at a later date was negative.

In December 2007, rising tumor markers led to imaging which prompted a biopsy of the right hip. This showed an estrogen receptor positive, progesterone receptor negative, HER2 negative tumor.

Femara was started in January 2008 and continued until progression in May 2015. Incidentally, disease control lasting seven years on letrozole is longer than anticipated for first line therapy for metastatic breast cancer. This is similar to several other women discussed in chapter 5.

Zometa began in 2008 to manage bone metastases. She has been on a Zometa holiday since January 2018.

At progression in June 2015, fulvestrant was started until July 2017 when a PET scan revealed liver lesions. Tamoxifen began in July 2017.

An MRI of the liver showed an increase in the size of a lesion in the left lobe and a liver biopsy was performed. It was 100% ER positive and 75% PR positive, and surprisingly, for the first time, the HER2 assay indicated HER2 positivity.

Tamoxifen was effective but discontinued in August 2017, to allow for a more aggressive clinical therapy approach. Taxotere, Herceptin, and Perjeta were started in August 2017, and a CT scan in October 2017 showed reduction in the size of the liver lesions.

After completion of six cycles of Taxotere, Herceptin, and Perjeta, which was complicated by severe Perjeta-related diarrhea, she began Aromasin and Herceptin in December 2017 in an effort to maintain a chemotherapy-induced remission. This was successful with good disease control for two years. However, in December 2019, progression in the liver was noted, and she was entered into a clinical trial with randomization to Kadcyla with or without tucatinib. As of March 2021, progression was again noted, and she started Enhertu.

Marlene has lived with MBC for thirteen years. Initially, the tumor was ER positive and HER2 negative, and she experienced good disease control for nine years on hormonal therapy alone (like the women in chapter 5).

Subsequently, the biology of the tumor changed to ER positive, HER2 positive, and she has been managed for the past four years with anti-HER2 strategies.

6, Marlene: Takeaway

Marlene was diagnosed with breast cancer twenty-seven years ago and has been treated for MBC for the past thirteen years. Her original tumor was estrogen-receptor positive, HER2 negative, as was her first recurrence. However, her recurrence in 2017 was triple positive. It is important to note that once metastasis is diagnosed, it cannot be taken for granted that it will have the same characteristics as the primary tumor. If Marlene's tumor had not been biopsied at the time of her second recurrence, we would not have known that it had mutated and was now HER2 positive.

As we have learned, it is important to biopsy metastases, but areas of caution must be interjected. Changes in biomarkers do occur, but interpretation of these changes is of critical importance. Many patients with breast cancer relapse in bone. Some of the chemicals used to separate bone from tumor are harsh (decalcification), and thus positive biomarkers can be degraded and become falsely negative. Great caution must be exercised when interpreting negative biomarkers results from a bone biopsy. If there is an option, always choose non-bone sites when possible, to avoid false negative bone biopsy results. If bone is to be biopsied, special techniques in specimen handling are necessary to preserve biomarker and genetic material.

Indeed, as we biopsy patients with MBC, we constantly see changes in the genomic makeup of these tumors as they progress. Thus, an oncologist will often repeat a biopsy and submit tissue or even blood samples for next-generation sequencing. These tests analyze the genetic makeup of each patient's tumor and can often direct patients to specific clinical trials that target individual mutations in a given patient's tumor. Such clinical trials are widely available across the country. Ask your doctor if you might benefit from this investigational approach.

In Marlene's case, tumor tissue was sent for next-generation sequencing. Interesting mutations were revealed. First, HER2 was detected by this technique further confirming her prior testing indicating HER2 positivity. Second, she was found to have a mutation in the P1K3CA gene. A new drug, alpelisib (Piqray), was approved to target this mutation. At the moment, the approval is limited to ER positive, HER2 negative tumors. Additionally, the benefit has only been confirmed in combination with fulvestrant, a drug Marlene had already received. However, now that it is approved, additional studies will be performed with this targeted therapy. At some point, this piece of information could become important in Marlene's care.

Marlene's Story

As I recount my breast cancer journey, it's unreal that this began in 1993. This is 2020, that's twenty-seven years ago!

I moved from Florida to California and was working as a nurse practitioner. I detected a small lump in my left breast.

After undergoing mammograms. I was advised to see a surgeon. I contacted Dr. Vogel, whom I knew from the University of Miami. I was only fifty years old, had breastfed my children, and had never taken a hormone. This could not be happening to me!

I followed Dr. Vogel's advice and saw the California physicians he recommended. In the end, my decision was to proceed with a double mastectomy and reconstruction. I saw a panel of breast cancer doctors who, because of size, ER and PR positivity status, and slow growth, recommended no further follow-up.

Remember, this was 1993. In 2007, I visited Dr. Vogel, mostly to say hello, as I was continually grateful for his advice.

As we spoke, he asked how I was feeling. I told him that I was fine other than a little pain in my right hip as a result of caring for my grandchildren. This tiny bit of information led him to order tumor markers which resulted in the diagnosis of metastatic disease.

The breast cancer then metastasized to my liver, and I began chemotherapy. It was then discovered that the HER2 status had changed from negative to positive, which happens in a small percentage of people. My therapy was changed to accommodate this change.

Today, I am enrolled in a research study, and I'm doing well. I consider myself a lucky person. I have lived a full and productive life with breast cancer. Also, I have had the guidance and care of such a knowledgeable and compassionate physician.

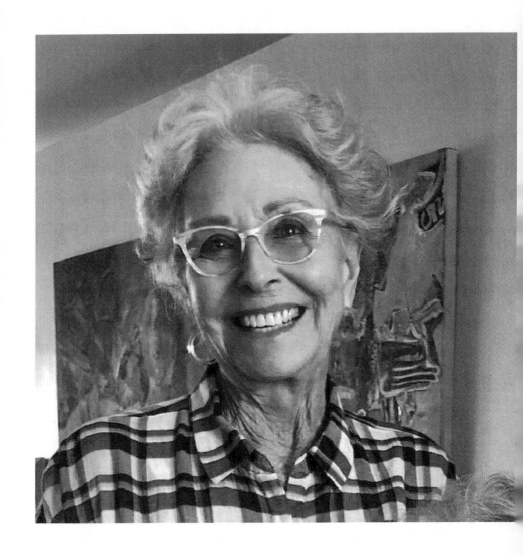

7: Georgia

In the fall of 2015, at age forty-five, Georgia was diagnosed with de novo stage 4 left breast cancer with a 6 cm breast tumor and bone metastases. Estrogen and progesterone receptors were negative, and HER2 was positive. Tumor markers were drawn. CA15-3 was elevated at 51, CEA was normal, and a PET scan identified lymph nodes under each arm and above the collarbone. The large breast mass was seen as well as multiple lesions throughout the spine and pelvis. Thus, the disease had spread to multiple areas in her body.

From November 2015 to February 2016, Georgia received Taxotere, Herceptin, and Perjeta and went into remission. In 2017, an MRI of the breast was completely normal. Since March 2016, she has only received Herceptin and Perjeta with no evidence of recurrence. She received Xgeva in the past, but it was discontinued due to possible osteonecrosis of the right foot. Although her overall remission at this point is only four and a half years, her response was remarkably good, and she continues to be without disease. We are hoping for a durable response and, who knows, maybe cure.

7, Georgia: Takeaway

Although still only four and a half years into remission of HER2 positive MBC it is after only an eighteen-week course of chemotherapy with the targeted therapy of Herceptin and Perjeta. Typically, for MBC that requires chemotherapy, the average duration of disease control is less than one year. The groundbreaking results of the Cleopatra trial (33) with Taxotere, Herceptin, and Perjeta given as first line treatment for HER2 positive MBC yielded extraordinary results, and Georgia benefitted from that advance. There are likely others on the Cleopatra trial who constitute a tail on the duration of the response curve. Like Georgia, such patients could start to wonder, *Dare I even think that perhaps I may have been cured?* Regardless, few such patients take a gamble to go off their maintenance Herceptin (with or without Perjeta). Some have gambled and come off Herceptin and appeared to have won (see chapter 7, "Andrea").

Georgia's Story

When I was a nurse in my early twenties, my work with the elderly gave me joy. To provide my service as a nurse and know that I was helping my patients by making their day a little brighter fulfilled me. I always tried to take a little extra time to sit and talk with my patients. The elderly love to reflect on their life experiences. As a young nurse at that time, I always felt blessed that my patients were able to open up and share with me. To this day, I treasure those talks. Those memories are filled with gratitude.

My core values of caring, love, hope, compassion, knowledge, spirituality, and friendship contributed to shape me as a nurse. As I progressed in my professional career and personal life, with changing roles throughout the years, these values became even more meaningful.

When I was diagnosed with HER2 positive metastatic breast cancer in October 2015 at the age of forty-five, I took on the dual role of patient and nurse. As a patient, I closely analyzed and managed the care I received for myself. From collaborating with my oncologist, fighting with my health insurer for timely authorizations for treatment and diagnostic testing, keeping myself healthy, and continuing to work full-time, I was both my own patient and my own nurse. Learning my weaknesses and strengths through the experience of illness and related grief has inspired me to further recognize the importance of gratitude.

Not one woman should feel alone when going through a breast cancer diagnosis. The stages of grief can be extremely difficult. Life, as I knew it, both ended and began with these simple but complex words: "You have breast cancer." In continuing with the values that I carry, an appreciation for gratitude is even more recognized than previously. What is meaningful to each of us is different. Our values are essential to how we want to live, share, and coexist with others, in turn, making each of us unique. With the simplicity of gratitude, what is meaningful can easily be found.

Your bone scan "lit up like a Christmas tree." Those were the exact words of the oncologist who initially diagnosed me with metastatic breast cancer. Stage 4 at the onset, he projected a life expectancy of three to nine months. Two years post diagnosis and chemotherapy every three weeks, I asked my oncologist specific questions related to survival and life expectancy. He did not have answers except to verbalize that Dr. Charles Vogel was *the* expert in HER2 disease. In my mind, I asked myself, "Why was I not with *the best*?" This very same day while receiving treatment, I called the University of Miami and set up an appointment with Dr. Vogel. That was November 2017, and now the time of this writing is November of 2020. Yes, Dr. Vogel is the best, and I trust his knowledge and expertise emphatically.

In living with metastatic breast cancer, at times, it is difficult to face adversity and hardship that coexists with the disease. Within adversity, strength appears. For women facing metastatic breast cancer, it is important to find an acceptance of adversity of grief during the experience of illness and move forward.

The stages of grief in an illness such as metastatic breast cancer are frightening and real. These unique emotions are both normal and common to experience when faced with a life-threatening illness. Careful management of acute and chronic grief emotions is extremely important. With the expression of the experience of illness through grief, the bridge to wellness can be found. By opening our hearts and minds, positive emotions can allow discovery and building of new skills, new ties, new knowledge, and new ways of being.

Hope sustains and motivates you to tap into your own capabilities and inventiveness to turn negatives into positives. It inspires you to plan for a better future, even after a diagnosis of HER2 metastatic disease. Having the confidence of being treated by Dr. Vogel is wonderful. He always makes his best effort and answers questions with evidence-based facts and honesty. For that, I have gratitude and consider him a blessing.

With the experiences of this diagnosis that I carry, today, an appreciation for gratitude is recognized moreover than previously. While what is meaningful to each of us is different, our values are essential to how we want to live, share, and coexist with a life-changing health challenge. With the simplicity of gratitude, even with a HER2-positive metastatic breast cancer diagnosis, a meaningful life can be found.

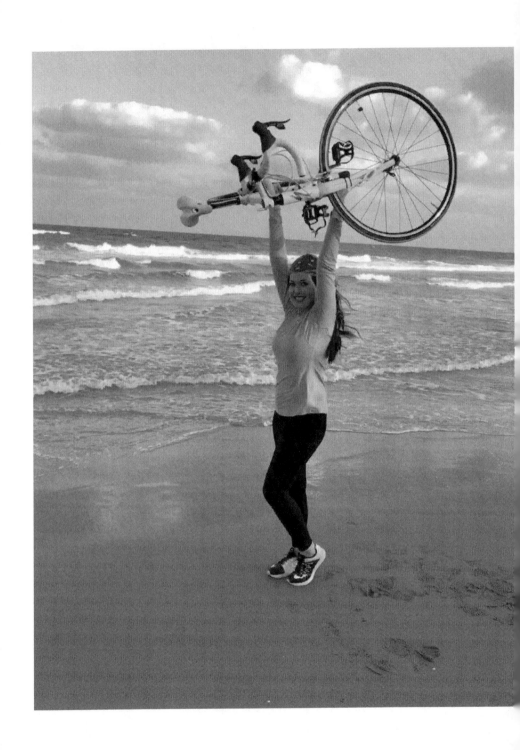

CHAPTER VII

HER2-Positive Pleomorphic Lobular Carcinoma

Introduction

Her2 positive pleomorphic lobular carcinoma is a very rare subtype of breast cancer. However, three of our patients with this diagnosis have had extraordinary clinical courses. How rare is this subtype in the United States? The approximate number of breast cancer patients in 2019 was 260,000. Lobular carcinoma constitutes 9% of all breast cancers, thus making 28,800 cases in 2019. Pleomorphic lobular carcinoma constitutes 33% of lobular carcinomas, which yields about 9,504 patients.

Pleomorphic lobular carcinomas that are HER2 positive constitute 33% of the pleomorphic lobular carcinomas. Therefore, about 3,136 patients were diagnosed with this rare subtype in 2019.

Given the rarity of this entity, we published a note in the *Journal of Clinical Oncology* calling attention to the extraordinary fact that three of our longer-term survivors have this rare form of breast cancer (36).

1: Beth

In early 1998, at thirty-eight years of age, Beth was diagnosed with left breast invasive lobular carcinoma and underwent a left mastectomy with fifteen of twenty lymph nodes positive. The diagnosis was pleomorphic lobular carcinoma, estrogen and progesterone negative, and HER2 positive.

Adriamycin and Cytoxan were delivered in the adjuvant setting, and a contralateral prophylactic mastectomy was also performed.

While receiving Cytoxan and Adriamycin, Beth experienced bone pain, and a bone scan showed bone metastases. She then transferred her medical care to our service.

Beginning in August 1998, she was treated with Xeloda, Aredia (an older bone-healing agent), and Herceptin. Thankfully, remission was induced by this regimen. Xeloda was continued for about eighteen months. She declined Xeloda discontinuation at six months and again at one year.

In January 2000, Beth began Herceptin alone. She also took the bisphosphonates Aredia and then Zometa for her bone metastases. Ultimately, I advised her to discontinue use in May 2011 due to stress fractures in her feet.

In spite of no evidence of cancer progression over the next twenty-two years, she has declined discontinuation of her every three weeks of Herceptin and continues to be disease-free.

1, Beth: Takeaway

This courageous young woman was diagnosed with HER2 positive disease prior to the FDA approval of Herceptin for treatment of MBC. At that time, the manufacturer of Herceptin (Genentech), with the advice of breast cancer advocates, instituted a lottery allowing patients chosen at random to receive the drug. Beth was one of those patients.

Why did we switch from the strong Adriamycin to Xeloda? Initially, Beth was treated with curative intent as she was not known to have metastatic disease. Once metastases were diagnosed, given the belief (still present in 2019) that metastatic disease is essentially not curable, the treatment philosophy changes to less toxic drugs. Although MBC is not curable, it is treatable, often with prolonged survival; hence, the rationale for this book.

Response to Xeloda and Herceptin was rapid, and thus, Beth's physicians tried to stop Xeloda on several occasions. Beth, having a very assertive personality, delayed discontinuation for eighteen months.

Beth elected to stay on bisphosphonate longer than her physician recommended. This class of drugs, which includes Zometa, Reclast, Boniva, Actonel, Fosamax, and others (including Aredia, which was one of the first intravenous bisphosphonates for bone metastases), when given for protracted periods of time, can lead to spontaneous fractures of bones. This complication is also seen with denosumab (Xgeva, Prolia), another bone-healing agent. After about five years of use, we began discussions to discontinue the Zometa. Beth declined initially. After eleven years of use, she developed stress fractures in her feet, and Zometa was discontinued.

Beth has no intention of going off Herceptin. Two other women in this chapter elected to stop Herceptin after thirteen and three and a half years respectively and remain disease-free. However, several others in this book, like Beth, continue on long-term Herceptin therapy. These authors personally believe that a subset of patients with HER2 positive disease may have been cured of metastatic disease. However, there are no meaningful data to support that belief other than anecdotal cases. Therefore, strong recommendations cannot be made for women like Beth who are disease-free for protracted periods of time. Beth has been disease-free for twenty-two years.

Beth's Story

Hi, my name is Beth, and I am a breast cancer thriver. I call myself a thriver because I have been living with stage 4 breast cancer for twenty-two years. I was diagnosed with breast cancer at age thirty-eight. It was a Sunday morning, and I remember feeling a lump in the shower. To be honest, I wasn't that concerned because I had very large breasts with lots of "lumps." A few years prior, I had one looked at by a surgeon, and it was just a cyst. For some reason, this lump felt different. On Monday, I called my gynecologist to evaluate the lump. At four o'clock the following Thursday, I got the call. I can remember it like it was yesterday. I was told that I had atypical cells and was recommended to see a surgeon. I didn't even know what atypical cells meant. I called my mom immediately and told her I had a lump, that the doctor said it had atypical cells, and that I needed to see a surgeon. She said, "You have breast cancer?" I said, "I'm really not sure yet." My life as I knew it changed forever that day.

At thirty-eight years old, my life was full. I was married to my best friend. I was a hairdresser and helped to run our plumbing company. Our two beautiful daughters were ten and twelve years old. You can imagine what was going through my mind when I got the diagnosis. I went into total survival mode. Immediately, my parents and I headed off to a cancer center in Miami to see the surgeon and confirm the diagnosis of breast cancer. They performed a biopsy in the office and confirmed that I had lobular breast cancer. They assured me I was in the right place and came up with a plan right away. No time to waste. I was sent across the street to the plastic surgeon's office to discuss reconstruction. All I remember is thinking to myself, *Please, God, get this cancer out of me so I can live and be there for my family.* I proceeded with a battery of tests, and the following week, I underwent a double mastectomy, followed by reconstruction.

I must admit, I knew nothing about breast cancer at the time. Boy did I get an education and quickly. The lump was not that large, but I had twenty lymph nodes taken out and fifteen were involved with cancer, so my cancer was aggressive. I was estrogen and progesterone negative. At that time, there was no test for HER2. Remember, it was twenty-two years ago. My treatment moved forward rather quickly. A port was placed in my chest, and within two weeks, I began chemotherapy. The planned schedule was to receive four rounds of chemo followed by a stem cell transplant. *Wow,* I survived chemo! Next, I was off to the plastic surgeon to exchange my expanders with permanent implants. At the time of the procedure, the surgeon could not believe what he found—cancer cells were growing. Needless to say, everyone was in shock. The chemo clearly did not work. Before additional recommendations could be made, I required imaging to determine if the cancer had spread. Unfortunately, it was discovered in my bones, and I was now stage 4. The stem cell transplant was called off and a new chemotherapy began. The doctors also wanted to try something novel, which was to radiate the left breast concurrently with chemotherapy. I agreed to this course of action. After all, I was young, strong, and had a will to do whatever was necessary to get rid of the cancer. To be honest, I'm sure I was only processing half of the information they were saying. All I wanted to do was stay alive.

During the chaos, with the help of my surgeon, I began my own research and discovered something they called HER2 and a drug called

Herceptin. I knew that somewhere in this world, there was an accurate test for HER2 because they were using it within a study. I insisted for Miami to send my tumor to be FISH tested. That test came back positive. I was on my second line of chemo treatments, and when that failed, I was offered to go into a lottery to get Herceptin. I started my third line of chemotherapy treatment waiting for my name to be pulled from the lottery. I had an angel on my shoulder because, two days later, I got the call! I was praying that this drug would work to slow the cancer and buy me time. After all, no chemotherapy seemed to be working. I received weekly infusions of Herceptin. Three months later, imaging showed that my disease was *stable*. My new favorite word. Till this day, twenty-two years later, I am still on Herceptin and stable. I thank God every day.

Not only was I diagnosed with stage 4 cancer, I also ended up with lymphedema in my left arm. To be honest, some days it is worse than the cancer. I deal with chronic cellulitis infections and ongoing lymphedema therapy to keep my arm from becoming as big as a leg. My nickname for my arm is Fat Arm. I have to laugh about it, or I'll cry. Can I say I hate my arm?

Through all of this, I have been blessed with a great support system. My mom and dad went to every treatment with me for many years. My husband rearranged his life and business to do whatever was necessary. I have a million friends who stepped in to help us out. I have a tremendous amount of faith, which I knew I needed to get through this. My church family prayed for me, along with people from all over the world. Just writing this, I get tears in my eyes. I feel so blessed that I am alive and that I was able to see my kids grow up. Being diagnosed with cancer taught me to be a much better person. I listen more, *really* listen. I was fortunate early on to have found a wonderful breast cancer group and became very involved within the breast cancer community. I wanted to give back. I became a patient advocate and also joined breast cancer groups online. When I was first diagnosed, one of the scariest things for me was the unknown. I put myself out there in hopes of helping others. I am always available to talk to patients and their families to support them any way I can. I've been involved in fundraising for Breast Cancer Research for many years because I believe research saves lives. My prayer is that everyone receives that magic drug that works for them.

At a very young age, I got my affairs in order. I planned my funeral and completed every bit of paperwork I could think of to make life easier for my husband and family—just in case. Then, I started to live. I must admit that living with cancer, I have really stepped out of my box. I have done things I might not have done if it wasn't for cancer. I know I am not guaranteed tomorrow and that anything could change. We live scan to scan. I love birthdays and getting older. "Keep counting up" is my motto. I am approaching twenty-three years, and my goal is to continue to create memories with everyone I love.

I know we are not supposed to mention our doctors, nurses, and radiologists, but they know I don't follow the rules very well, LOL. With the grace of God and my A-team, I am here and thriving. They have become my friends and family over the years. We are growing old together. Let's keep counting *up*.

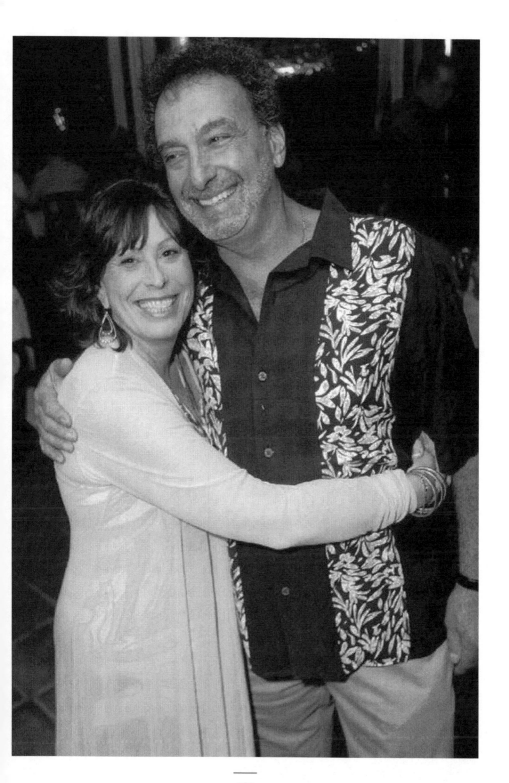

2: Andrea

Andrea was diagnosed in 1995 at age fifty-three with ER and PR positive breast cancer. She underwent a left mastectomy, and positive axillary nodes were discovered. Details of her initial treatment protocol are unavailable.

She did well until 1998 when she developed liver metastases. She received Adriamycin, then CMF chemotherapy, and subsequently docetaxel as a single agent. Herceptin was added after two months and continued for ten years. The docetaxel was discontinued after six doses.

Her oncologist began discussions of discontinuation of Herceptin after a few years of successful therapy. Finally, in 2008 Andrea, an intelligent free thinker, decided to discontinue Herceptin while in remission.

Andrea remains in remission thirteen years later on no antineoplastic therapy after the diagnosis of MBC to the liver twenty-three years ago earlier.

2, Andrea: Takeaway

At several points in this book, we have alluded to the conundrum of MBC patients with HER2-positive tumors who have experienced long, durable remissions but continue Herceptin for many years (see chapter 6, "Pat," or "Georgia"; chapter 8, "Kelly"; chapter 3, "Patricia"; chapter 7, "Beth").

Andrea was one of the few who have gambled that, perhaps, there is a cure for some patients with HER2-positive MBC. Andrea remains disease-free twenty-three years after the diagnosis of MBC to the liver and thirteen years after stopping Herceptin.

3: Jean

Jean was diagnosed with pleomorphic lobular carcinoma and underwent a right mastectomy in August 2004 at age fifty-five. No lymph nodes were involved, but she was HER2 positive. ER and PR were negative. She elected to have a left prophylactic mastectomy without reconstruction.

She received adjuvant therapy with dose dense AC followed by Taxol. She did well for less than two years and relapsed in May 2006 when a vertebral biopsy indicated cancer.

Chemotherapy with Navelbine and Herceptin was delivered from March 2006 until April 2006 with poor tolerance of Navelbine. She then received single agent Herceptin until September 2009 when she again relapsed. Jean began an investigational protocol with TDM1 (Kadcyla) plus pertuzumab (Perjeta) for an enlarging mass in the left adrenal gland. She also had bone metastases and therefore started on Zometa that was poorly tolerated and discontinued.

In January 2018, she came off all therapy due to neuropathy.

Jean received Herceptin for three years and then Perjeta with Kadcyla for twelve years. However, for the past three and a half years, she has been on no systemic therapy for her previous diagnosis of MBC and remains disease-free at this time.

Jean's Long and Winding Road: 2004 to 2020

2004

I was first diagnosed with breast cancer in August 2004 at the age of fifty-four. I received a phone call from my breast surgeon telling me that I was on his "VIP List"—a list that you really don't want to be on. I was diagnosed with ductal carcinoma in situ, but he said I should not be overly worried as this type of noninvasive breast cancer is most times 100% curable with a lumpectomy. I visited him the next day, and he ordered additional confirmatory tests and referred me to reconstructive surgeons. My husband, Michael, and I breathed a sigh of relief.

Almost unbelievably, I ran into my thirty-four-year-old next-door neighbor in the waiting room. She told me that she, too, was just diagnosed with breast cancer and was a patient of the same doctor. A couple of days later, I underwent a breast MRI. The day after the MRI, I received a call that additional imaging was necessary. When I arrived at the women's center, I was met by a doctor who told me that they needed some tissue. I asked her, "Why all of the fuss?" as I had been diagnosed with DCIS and was scheduling imminent surgery. "Oh no," she said, "you were diagnosed with invasive breast cancer." I was in shock. I was never contacted by my breast doctor after the MRI. I was confused and scared. After arriving home and sharing the bad news with Michael, we called my doctor, who apologized that he had not called me earlier. Given my age and family history, I scheduled a bilateral mastectomy along with a sentinel node biopsy. Life was hectic and flying by. Our college freshman daughter was selected to compete on a TV reality show for large cash prizes. Major hurricanes seemed to be predicted every two weeks. Finally, I underwent my surgery. My surgeon spoke to Michael directly after the surgery and informed him that, thankfully, I was node negative—but the full nodal pathology had to come back to confirm this. After waking up from surgery, we received a phone call from our college freshman daughter to share that she had just won $77,000 on a game show! What a turn of events! My perspective started to turn more positive.

We visited the surgeon for pathology results. He reported that the nodal pathology was completely negative and said that the chance of further spread was almost nil. "You have a 99% chance of no further spread." Michael and I both had tears of joy at this news, although he cautioned us that given the size and type of tumor that had been removed, I would still require chemotherapy. My attitude was super positive. I met with an oncologist who told me that I was diagnosed as triple negative using the IHC test, which meant there were virtually no drugs other than standard chemo he could prescribe. He put me through bi-weekly intensified therapy known in those days as ACT: Adriamycin, Cytoxan, and Taxol. I did not tolerate chemotherapy well and became very ill. However, I took my treatment with my next-door neighbor, and it made things much easier to deal with psychologically. I knew that I was not alone and could not feel sorry for myself as this young woman with two young children was going through the same thing as me. Her cancer had a worse prognosis than mine. However, as the weeks passed, I started to fear dying, mainly from the effects of the chemo. I lost my hair and a great deal of weight. I experienced extreme fatigue. I decided to go off therapy early due to the side effects, and most importantly, because I was node negative, I believed chemo was not worth the side effects.

2005

I recovered quickly after stopping chemo, and my hair grew back over a couple of months. I gained weight and traveled with friends. Life was good. In September 2005, while I was out to dinner with my neighbor celebrating a year from our surgery, Michael received a call from my oncologist indicating that my routine tumor markers had just come back with a significant upward spike. When I returned home that evening, he could not bring himself to tell me. When I awoke the next morning and saw his exhausted face, I knew there was something wrong. He told me about the phone call, and we went to the oncologist that morning for additional lab work. We received the bad news that afternoon: the tumor markers were even higher. My cancer had returned and spread; it was now incurable. Days of testing revealed the cancer involved my bones; my scans lit up like a Christmas tree. Unbeknownst to me, my oncologist took Michael aside and told him that I likely had just a few months left. Michael never told me this until years later. The odd thing, however, was that I felt great physically. The next day, Michael took me golfing to get my mind off things. During the round, I hit the ground with my club and felt a painful crack in my chest. I had broken a rib. That coming week, I saw a well-known geneticist to discuss testing for the BRCA gene. While waiting to see her, Michael was passing time by reading my quite extensive medical folder, which the geneticist's assistant had left on the table. All of sudden, he turns and says to me, "Jean, this report says that you overexpress HER2 protein at a very high level." At that moment, the geneticist comes into the room. We showed her the report, and after some digging, she finds out that my tissue had been entered into a randomized validation of a new pathology test called the FISH test. This huge change in diagnosis was only discovered by the happenstance of Michael thumbing through my file. No one had contacted me or my oncologist. The next day, I saw Dr. Charles Vogel, a trailblazer in the use of Herceptin as a treatment. He read the report and immediately prescribed Herceptin treatment for me, which began quickly. Within a couple of months, my scans showed "No Evidence of Disease" (NED). I would live.

2009

After switching to Dr. Vogel as my oncologist in early 2006, I remained on Herceptin with no perceivable side effects for three years. In 2009, a routine scan revealed that the cancer had returned in my adrenal gland. I remember Dr. Vogel telling us that the cancer was "breaking through." However, he also told us that there was a new clinical trial showing fantastic results in patients for whom Herceptin had stopped suppressing the cancer. It was called TDM1. It took a while to get me into the trial using TDM1 and another drug, Pertuzumab. Due to the various onco-politics involved in trials, I had to travel to Philadelphia to receive treatment every three weeks. After about a year, I was able to participate in the same trial locally in Florida. I tolerated the stronger drugs, but experienced neuropathy, balance issues, and weight loss—problems, but nothing like chemo. I fell three times as a result of balance issues. Due to injuries, I eventually underwent a second knee replacement. I also cracked my head open when I fell and hit a piece of furniture. Still, I persevered. I remained on the trial until January 2018, when I determined that after nine years of NED, it was time to take a break. The TDM1 is now FDA approved and is called Kadcyla. Pertuzumab is approved and is called Perjeta. My surviving was a major reason for proving its success—and that is a wonderful feeling for me.

2020

It is now 2020, and my side effects are nearly gone, my weight has returned to normal, and I am no longer falling over after losing my balance. I have received no further therapy since January 2018, and my CAT scans in June 2020 were negative. I feel oddly honored and lucky to have gone through this entire experience, both good and bad. Spending years in chemo chairs, hour after hour watching women younger than me go through this process no longer feels like a chore; it feels like redemption. My minor suffering has helped future generations of women, and for that I am grateful. Best of all, my young neighbor, who was diagnosed with triple-negative cancer also went on a clinical trial and is still doing great after sixteen years. But there is one thing for sure: Charles Vogel saved my life. My advice to newly diagnosed patients is to be proactive! Question everything, push the limits, and never give up. Cancer treatment today is far ahead of where it was when I was first diagnosed. Whether you know it or not, we are biological warriors for our daughters and granddaughters. Whatever we suffer will help untold millions of women in the future. Use the rest of your life to enjoy yourself; I know I am. Don't waste time feeling sorry for yourself. Don't waste time worrying about what you can't control. In my mind, I have already won—any time I have left now is gravy.

2 and 3, Andrea and Jean: Takeaway

First, both of these women, like Beth (chapter 7) had a relatively rare variant of MBC, pleomorphic lobular carcinoma, with all three having protracted outcomes with MBC (twenty two, twenty three, and fifteen years, respectively). This could be coincidence or could point to some protein or gene common to all suggesting profound sensitivity to Herceptin.

Beth, like others in this book (chapter 4, Patricia; chapter 6, Pat), has chosen to continue Herceptin indefinitely, while Andrea and Jean are hoping that, indeed, there may be a cure for some women with MBC.

Likely, there are hundreds of such patients put into dramatic remissions of HER2 positive breast cancer. They are now experiencing protracted remissions wondering whether or not, at some point, they can stop this medicine and hope that "I have been cured" (21).

Chapter VIII

HER2-Positive Disease with Brain Metastases

Introduction

HER2-positive metastatic breast cancer patients are at high risk for developing brain metastases with greater than 30% of the patients developing lesions in the brain. (37,38). As patients live longer due to more effective systemic therapy, the incidence of brain metastases is increasing. Up to 80% of women who develop metastatic disease ultimately develop brain lesions with an average time to progression of 13.3 months (37). Risk factors associated with development of CNS (central nervous system) metastases are age <50, ER/PR-negative disease, 3 or more sites of disease or recurrent MBC.

American Society of Clinical Oncology (ASCO) has developed guidelines for management of brain metastases in HER2-positive patients (39).

Many of the systemic therapies available do not cross the blood-brain barrier, and this is a significant challenge in the management of brain lesions. Herceptin is not thought to cross the blood-brain barrier. Newer therapy, called tyrosine kinase inhibitors (TKI), Tykerb, neratinib, and tucatinib are being investigated as they show better blood-brain-barrier penetration. Specifically, neratinib, is promising for being effective in patients with brain metastases who are HER2 positive. When given with the drug capecitabine, responses in the central nervous system were between 30 and 50% as noted on a study (40). A randomized controlled study that used the drug neratinib with capecitabine showed that patients with this regimen experienced improvement in one-year progression-free survival with the cumulative incidence of CNS metastases being lower as compared to Tykerb in combination with capecitabine (41). The side effect of diarrhea associated with neratinib has been a challenge and is an issue.

Another TKI, tucatinib, is promising in the field and selectively targets HER2. In one study, patients received the drug with trastuzumab and capecitabine. The patients had already received a number of other treatments for metastatic disease (42). Patients had improvement in progression-free survival. There was a 52% reduction in patients with brain metastases in terms of risk of progression or death. Therefore, these patients did much better with regards to the brain-related issues. Of note, diarrhea was much less of an issue. Of the patients who did develop brain metastases in this trial, the patients who received tucatinib did much better. These patients had a better response in the brain and had a decrease in the progression in the brain or death from CNS issues, as well as improvement in survival (43).

While systemic therapy continues to improve with regards to CNS disease, the mainstay of brain metastases treatment is typically radiation, which is known to shrink tumors. When the number of tumors in the brain is small, targeted treatment (Gamma Knife or stereotactic brain radiation) may be delivered, which is less toxic to the surrounding normal brain. When the disease is more diffuse, whole brain radiation is the optimal treatment, as it will cover all areas of concern.

Studies have shown that deterioration in thought processes at six months is less frequent in patients treated with targeted brain radiation as compared to whole brain radiation without a change in overall survival (44). This is very important for patients, as memory and thought processing is important for quality of life.

An additional tool for minimizing deterioration in thought processes is a medication that can be given along with brain radiation. This is called memantine and is a drug used for Alzheimer's patients. Patients who took this drug with whole brain radiation had a significantly longer time to memory decline and also had better results in testing in terms of executive function, processing speed, and delayed recall (45). It is relatively well tolerated.

Also, fancy radiation planning can help with memory as well. A special technique that avoids the part of the brain responsible for memory, the hippocampus, can be utilized if no brain lesions are near this area. When compared to traditional whole brain radiation, patients with hippocampal avoidance had a significantly lower risk of memory failure when treated with memantine (46). There was no difference in overall survival or the chances of progressing in the brain; however, the patients with the specialized treatment had less difficulty remembering things, less difficulty speaking, and fewer cognitive symptoms.

The advances noted above including targeted radiation to just the tumors, whole brain radiation avoiding the neurocognitive portion of the brain, memantine, and the newer systemic agents are allowing patients to have better outcomes in the setting of HER2-positive metastatic cancer with brain metastases.

1: Lisa

At diagnosis in 2010, Lisa was forty-three years old. She was discovered to have cancer in both breasts. One was triple negative and one was HER2 positive but estrogen and progesterone negative.

She received AC followed by Taxol but, initially, no Herceptin was given for unclear reasons. However, Herceptin was added after Taxol. This is compatible with the sequential use of chemotherapy followed by Herceptin in the adjuvant setting in the European HERA trial (see Lisa's "Take Home Message").

Lisa did well until 2011 when she developed a lung metastasis that was triple negative. It was surgically removed with no additional therapy given.

In August 2012, Lisa developed a liver lesion that was biopsied and found to be breast cancer that was HER2 positive but ER and PR negative. She took Taxotere, Herceptin, and Perjeta until November 2012. At that time, Taxotere was discontinued after six doses. There was no cancer seen on imaging. Herceptin and Perjeta continued from 2013 to the present time in June 2021 (nine-plus years).

Unfortunately, in December 2014, while on Herceptin and Perjeta, Lisa developed brain metastases. They were discovered on an MRI scan after she noted difficulty with gait.

Lisa underwent surgical removal of the largest tumor, and eight days after the procedure, Lisa and her fiancé were married. She walked down the aisle as a beautiful bride.

Lisa required whole brain radiation and entered a clinical trial randomizing between brain radiation alone or in combination with a short course of Tykerb (another anti-HER2 systemic drug). Lisa was randomized to brain radiation alone.

Lisa was maintained on Herceptin and Perjeta every three weeks starting in 2012.

In September 2019, she underwent robotic assisted removal of an isolated mediastinal lymph node that was ER negative and HER2 positive cancer, followed by radiation therapy to the surgical bed. This was the only area of recurrence, and she continues on the same systemic therapy. As of February 2021, Lisa remains disease-free. She is experiencing issues related to postradiation effects including difficulty with gait. She continues full-time employment.

Lisa has had breast cancer for eleven years, MBC for ten years, brain metastases seven years earlier, and has been on Herceptin and Perjeta for nine-plus years with her last chemotherapy nine years ago.

1, Lisa: Takeaway

It is possible to have different tumors in each breast like Lisa, but patients may also have different tumors in the same breast. When these tumors have different phenotypes (ER, PR, and HER2 neu), it is called heterogeneity.

At diagnosis, Lisa should have been treated with AC followed by concomitant Taxol plus Herceptin, which would have covered both her triple-negative and HER2-positive cancers. Herceptin clinical trials have shown that concomitant chemotherapy plus Herceptin is superior to the Hera approach of sequential therapy (47).

As noted, Lisa had two different primary tumors. She had a triple negative tumor in one breast and a hormone receptor negative but HER2 positive tumor in the other. When she first experienced a relapse, it was a triple-negative tumor in the lung. Her second relapse was with a HER2 positive tumor in her liver. This reminds us of the importance of a biopsy at the time of recurrence. In Lisa's situation, it relates to the differences of her two different primary tumors. In other patients, it is because the hormonal and HER2 receptors may have changed to a different subtype from the original tumor at the time of relapse (see chapter 6, "Marlene").

HER2 positive tumors have a strong propensity to spread to the brain. In Lisa's case, after optimal neurosurgical care and continuing care by radiation oncology, control was achieved and, to date, continues.

Appropriate treatment of HER2-positive metastases can lead to long and sometimes extraordinarily protracted metastatic control. Lisa, has continued on Herceptin and Perjeta for eight-plus years after diagnosis of lung, brain and liver metastases.

Not only is Lisa an extremely brave and beautiful young woman but walking down the aisle to marry her love eight days after brain surgery showed *true grit*.

Lisa's Story

In May of 2020, I reached the ten-year anniversary of my diagnosis with breast cancer. I am a wife, a mom, a daughter, a sister, a friend, and a full-time office administrator for a busy law firm. In the past ten years, I have been blessed with a proposal and marriage and had the privilege of and seeing my children and stepchildren graduate from high school and college to become adults with great ambition and achievements in their lives. We are a family scattered all over, with people living in Tampa; Denver; Fairfax, Virginia; Japan; and Tallahassee. Over the past ten years, we have traveled to Aruba, Argentina, Cancun, and Japan, as well as various trips around the United States to visit family and friends.

Looking back on this journey is the only way to keep looking forward. The Friday before Mother's Day in 2010, I was forty-three years old and a single mother of three children: Kara, seventeen at the time, had just graduated high school and would be starting college at Florida State University. Brennan, my son, was thirteen and finishing eighth grade; and Ally, nine years old, was finishing fifth grade. They were my world, and I was happily dating my future husband, Todd.

I had lumps in both breasts nine months prior, but the breast surgeon who reviewed my mammogram said they were cysts and to come back in nine months. My mother had cystic breasts, and so this was great news, and life went on for a few months. But it turned out the breast surgeon was wrong.

My dear friend's husband is an oncologist, and he ordered a biopsy after I complained about pain in my breasts. The biopsy confirmed that I had breast cancer, and I started chemotherapy within a week. I was afraid but stayed strong for my kids and said lots of prayers, mostly about being able to finish raising them. I wanted their lives to be carefree and for them to know I would get through this and be OK. I also worked full-time during chemotherapy. I would leave work after a half day on Friday, have chemotherapy, recover over the weekend, and return to work on Monday. Breast cancer was not going to change my life; it would have to work around me.

My parents and my community rallied around me. So many random acts of kindness filled my life. I was not in this alone. To my dismay, even my son shaved his head so that I was not the only bald person at home. Why would he do this before his eighth-grade graduation?

After seeing a second breast surgeon after chemotherapy to prepare for mastectomy, it was noted that I had two different types of breast cancer. Only one breast tumor was biopsied, and it was triple negative, but the second tumor was HER2 positive. This led to a full year of Herceptin after I finished chemotherapy. I also underwent a bilateral mastectomy and radiation. Herceptin is a miracle drug, and I am still on it today.

My journey with breast cancer has been challenging at times, but I would not let it define me as a person. I did not have time for cancer because there was too much to do and get done—too many memories to make! These included events such as Mom's weekend at FSU, baseball games, and cheer competitions. I was blessed with great kids, love and support from family and friends, and many prayers. I was not alone. My husband always used the words "We will get through this," and my parents became my kids' chaperone to doctor and dentist appointments, my help with lawn and garden workers, and maintenance people. At the time, my husband lived in another state but fortunately was able to sit with me at treatments and love me through all that went along with battling cancer.

It did not take long for my first metastasis to appear; it was in the upper right lobe of my lung. I sought an opinion with Dr. Vogel at the Sylvester Cancer Center, as my breast surgeon had highly recommended him. A small section of my lung was removed, and I was sent home a day later, but not without a quick stop at my son Brennan's baseball game. No further treatment was needed. My hair grew back, and my kids called it baby duck hair. I was feeling well. I finally had a full head of short hair, and then I was diagnosed with a spot on my liver. I went to MD Anderson for a biopsy and evaluation, and, oh no, more chemotherapy. Fortunately, the chemotherapy took care of the cancer in the liver, and no other treatment or surgery was necessary.

For round 2 of chemo, my nurse gave me information on cold caps, which minimize hair loss. It was a tough process, but after completion of chemotherapy, I still had hair. It was scraggly hair, but it was hair, and it was worth it. I was living with stage 4 breast cancer. I was living a wonderful and productive life, and I had hair!

Then, I experienced difficulty navigating stairs. I thought I had vertigo. However, after notifying Dr. Vogel of my symptoms, I underwent a STAT MRI, and I was diagnosed with a 3 cm metastasis in the right side of my brain. Oddly, I was not afraid. I had faith, and I knew it was going to be OK. We met with the surgeon, and less than a week later, the tumor was removed—just ten days before our wedding day. The surgeon did his best to work around my hair. I was married with my brother officiating, our children by our side, and closest friends and family with us. After a few weeks of healing, I started whole brain radiation. I was stable for five years with IV treatments every three weeks.

My most recent metastasis was a small spot behind my chest wall. My medical team had watched this spot for many years, and it changed slightly, so it was removed and then treated with radiation. I was not afraid.

I am blessed. I am strong. I am proud to share my journey with you and others who are afraid and worried about what is to come. I have had ten years of joy, and I plan on many more. I am a perfect example that you can live with stage 4 breast cancer. You can be a wife, a mother, a daughter, a caregiver, and a friend. I fought cancer and won every time with the help of my doctors, nurses, and the amazing team at Sylvester Comprehensive Cancer Center.

My life currently is very exciting. Recently, Todd's daughter Carlye gave us the gift of becoming grandparents to a beautiful baby girl. We have the upcoming wedding of my daughter, Kara. Todd's son Blake settled in Denver and loves working for a major airline, and my son, Brennan, just became a first lieutenant in the air force. Finally, Ally is starting her sophomore year at FSU with plans to become a physical therapist. I am married to my best friend and protector, who brings me flowers every treatment day. Life is good.

My doctors and nurses have become my friends. I am blessed, and I am not afraid.

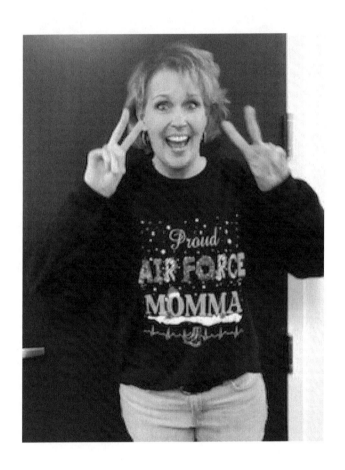

2: Kirsten

At age thirty-four in October 2010, Kirsten underwent a left lumpectomy and radiation therapy for a 1.4 cm grade 2 invasive ductal carcinoma that was triple positive.

Taxol and Herceptin were given, and she completed one year of Herceptin in February 2012. She wanted to consider pregnancy and thus declined recommended tamoxifen.

In February 2013, Kirsten was noted to have elevated tumor markers. This led to diagnosis of metastatic disease to lymph nodes and liver.

She received therapy on the Velvet Clinical Trial with Navelbine, Herceptin, and Perjeta from May 2013 to July 2015 with an excellent response, even after Navelbine was stopped. She continued Herceptin and Perjeta but went off study in March of 2017.

While on Herceptin and Perjeta, in August of 2015, Kirsten experienced a seizure. MRI of the brain showed two lesions including a large right parietal lesion and a smaller focus in the right frontal lobe.

She underwent resection of the right parietal metastasis and subsequently underwent Gamma Knife radiation to the tumor bed and to the second lesion in September 2015. Pathology from the brain tumor was consistent with the breast primary. It was HER2 positive and focally positive for estrogen receptor and also progesterone receptor positive.

In April 2017, there was slight systemic progression, and thus Kirsten began Kadcyla. It continued until August 2018 when it was discontinued due to low blood counts. Since August 2018, Kirsten has been maintained solely on Herceptin.

Kirsten has had breast cancer for eleven years, MBC for eight years, and was treated for brain metastases six years ago.

2, Kirsten: Takeaway

As of March 2021, Kirsten works full time, recently won the Palm Beach version of *Dancing with the Stars* and appears to be living a normal life with controlled liver and brain metastases. Beneath the surface, however, every three weeks Herceptin and every three to six months scans and echocardiograms weigh heavily on her emotionally. As with all patients living with MBC, there are intermittent but constant reminders that the other shoe could drop at any time.

Fortunately, since Kirsten's diagnosis of MBC eight years ago, there have been numerous therapy advances with many more on the horizon. Within the past year, neratinib, tucatinib, Enhertu, and margetuximab have all been approved. At least two of those have shown activity in brain metastases.

Although no one can predict the future, even if that other shoe does drop, there are many promising treatments that can help keep Kirsten the highly functional professional and loving wife for years to come.

Kirsten's Story

I have stage 4 breast cancer. Since my original diagnosis in 2010, I have juggled a full-time job, multiple volunteer roles, and family obligations with chemotherapy, radiation, and surgical procedures. Every morning when I look in the mirror, I realize that I am the face of cancer. I am also reminded that I am the reflection of many women's worst fears. It was not something that could ever happen to me, and yet it did.

Ultimately, I am open about the cancer to help myself. Yet this openness requires a thick skin. Early on, an acquaintance taught me that we still have a long way to go to understand how to support each other through a cancer diagnosis. We continue to struggle with how to share our expertise.

I can vividly recall eating a cupcake at an event when a woman came up to me and mentioned that the sugar I was eating was feeding my cancer. Lucky for her, she said this just as I had shoved the entire cupcake in my mouth. My first urge was to get another one and shove it in her face. My second urge was to say something mean, but my full mouth and lack of wit saved me from an inappropriate comeback. With time, I learned that in general, diet can be important, but the one mini cupcake wasn't going to kill me. I was defensive because I felt she was judging me.

In spite of recognizing this, I note that I judge others. I remember feeling so angry knowing that a friend had two healthy children after years of heroin abuse. I was living a nightmare but had lived a clean lifestyle; the worst things that I had done was drink wine and eat dessert. Seeing her boys brought forth emotions I had never really known envy and resentment. Over time, I have come to believe her children are an example of how the body has a tremendous capability to heal itself.

The mind, however, takes a long time to recover. I once believed that if I set my mind to it, I could do anything. I now know that there are times when it no longer matters how hard I work. What I want most is not achievable.

In 2013, I lost my engagement ring, the rock that literally got me though my first rounds of chemo. Less than a week later, I was standing in my front yard desperately hugging my husband, feeling his heart race as I told him the cancer was back and had metastasized to my lymph nodes and liver. All I could feel was rage against the body that betrayed me and the god that abandoned me.

Three months later, I received a phone call from a research nurse stating that a blood test indicated I was pregnant. After a night of agony struggling with what this news meant to me and the decisions I would face, I was told there had been a "lab error," something that never happens. There are things I have had to bury deep in order to get out of bed in the morning and to be around people who remind me of a time when my life had endless promise.

However, being around people and being a part of a community is essential to healing, as is humor. My husband uses humor to help me face my fears and accept drastic changes to my body. When I had a lumpectomy, it was followed by a week of internal radiation in my left breast. When the bandages were removed, I was terrified of the deformity I would encounter. When I asked Tom how bad it was, he told me the left one looked better than the right. To use his words, "the left was high and tight" from all the radiation. I immediately ran to the mirror. His remarks weren't exactly accurate, but it wasn't as awful as I had envisioned. Ten years later, that scar is barely visible.

I have learned to laugh in tough times. I have also learned to keep going and to stay connected and maintain a sense of compassion. With every scan and setback, I receive, I choose my reaction. I live with a statistical reality that I only have a 20% chance of survival five years post metastasis. As I write this, I am on year 7 post diagnosis of metastatic disease. I choose not to live within the confines of this diagnosis. I have every reason to be mad or overwhelmed. To survive, I have to respond to each challenge with an attitude of how do I positively move forward? I also have to understand that I have people in my life who will do anything to help me. I am blessed with unconditional love and unwavering support.

On August 20, 2015, I had just returned to work from a lunch when I couldn't move my left arm. I stood and I couldn't move my left leg. After literally dragging myself out of my office trying to be discreet. Tom had to literally carry me from the bottom of the stairs outside my office to my car and then into the ER.

Subsequent scans revealed two malignant brain tumors. Within three days, I was able to get in to see a world-renowned brain surgeon (who happened to be a year behind me at Duke, which caused its own anxiety) I remember thinking he can't have that much practice since I can't be that old. Initially, we were looking at surgery a week out, but considering a tropical system in the Atlantic, I pushed him for an earlier date, which happened to be the next day. After running my mouth, I was told I was not leaving the hospital. Yet twenty-four hours later, I was home and back at work the following Monday.

Battling breast cancer, the disease, and even more so its treatments has challenged my dignity and sense of self: my hair has fallen out in clumps, my brain and my breasts have been scarred and subjected to radiation, and my fertility has been destroyed.

When I was first diagnosed, I was told to have some eggs retrieved as an "insurance policy." Every January, I paid the storage bill for the three eggs, with hope that it would be the year a miracle would happen, and I wouldn't need the policy. But my miracle never came. Years after I finally accepted that I could never carry my own children and feeling certain that Tom was 200% committed to raising any children alone, we pursued surrogacy. Having the eggs on ice gave me hope. After thirteen false starts with various surrogates (each false start its own cruel story), we were able to implant two eggs. The call a few weeks later that the surrogate wasn't pregnant was the worst news of my life, and this is coming from someone who faced brain surgery. I went into a depression that I am still not sure I have fully recovered from.

You never know what is going on beneath the surface. I am the picture of health and can play tennis for three and half hours, yet I experience bleeding from my gums because my platelet counts were at all-time lows. It would be so easy to succumb to jealousy and rage as my body continues to betray me.

To survive, I respond to each disappointment the only way I know—to work harder and raise the bar on my cognitive and physical abilities. I don't know what tomorrow will bring, but with each tomorrow that I get, I am beating the odds.

3: Kelly

At age forty-six, in October 2005, Kelly was diagnosed with a left breast invasive ductal carcinoma with lymph nodes involved. The tumor was ER and PR negative and HER2 positive. She received neoadjuvant chemotherapy with AC for one dose and then TCH for four cycles from November 2005 to February 2006. This was followed by continuation of Herceptin until May 2006.

In March 2006, Kelly underwent a left breast lumpectomy which showed a pathologic complete response in the breast and lymph nodes. There was no remaining cancer.

Postoperatively, she began Adriamycin and Cytoxan, but it was stopped after one dose, as she could not tolerate the side effects

Comprehensive breast and nodal radiation was completed in July 2006.

In May 2007, Kelly had an isolated brain metastasis discovered after noting significant elevations of a tumor marker, CEA. No other systemic disease was identified. The brain tumor was treated with Gamma Knife radiation.

Tykerb, as a single agent, was started in June 2007. Kelly underwent Gamma Knife radiation in April 2008 for another brain lesion. Later in December, she was found to have a third brain tumor, and Xeloda was added after another gamma knife. She has been on Xeloda with Tykerb since that time with minimal toxicity.

As of March 2021, Kelly has no symptoms related to breast cancer or her brain metastases and is tolerating Xeloda and Tykerb quite well. She has been disease-free since the treatment of her brain metastases in 2008 (now 14 years disease free as of 2022.)

3, Kelly: Takeaway

Kelly's story is unique in several regards. First, *all* of Kelly's issues with MBC have been in the brain.

Second, all of her brain lesions were managed by Gamma Knife, highly localized radiation therapy. She did not have surgical intervention on her brain. She has not required whole brain radiation therapy which can be associated with long-term, troubling side effects.

Third, Kelly has been maintained on a combination of lapatinib (Tykerb) and Xeloda for fourteen years without toxicity. Thus, Kelly faces the conundrum we have mentioned several times in this book. After thirteen years, dare Kelly hope that she may actually have been cured of her brain metastases and stop these drugs, like Andrea (chapter 7)?

Finally, for select patients, lapatinib has been a wonder drug. With the advent of neratinib and tucatinib, lapatinib is falling toward the back of the line in therapeutic options. However, for some, like Kelly and Karen (chapter 8), it has been a lifesaver.

Kelly's Story

My name is Kelly, and my journey began in the summer of 2005, at the age of forty-six. My family and I were vacationing in Michigan, and my husband and I were excited to take our eldest daughter, Brooke, to college that fall. Our youngest daughter, Brittany, was going to start her junior year in high school. During this family vacation, my husband found a lump in my left breast. My medical insurance did not cover me while out of state. Thus, I had to wait until I returned to Florida for an ultrasound and needle biopsy Once that was done, the wait continued.

In September, I got the call no one wants to receive. The doctor advised me that the results showed cancer.

I knew then that I needed to find the best oncologist, so I did research and spoke with several people who had cancer, and they recommended Dr. Vogel. I made an appointment to see Dr. Vogel and his recommendation was chemotherapy followed by lumpectomy. Being the type of person I am, I sought a second opinion at Moffitt Cancer Center. Dr. Vogel understood and personally sent an email to the head breast surgeon with a recommendation for a lumpectomy with an incisional biopsy to find out exactly what type and stage cancer we were dealing with.

I went to Moffitt and underwent the biopsy and had a port placed. I then returned home to Coral Springs to await results.

The results decided to come in the week Hurricane Wilma hit Broward County, and everything was closed. My tumor was ER and PR negative and HER2 positive. I wanted to start my treatment right away as my husband was beside himself, and my daughters were very distraught.

I called Dr. Vogel to ask if I could go to Tampa to start chemotherapy. He agreed that I could go there to start. However, it was critical to verify the chemotherapy.

My husband and I drove to the Moffitt Center I received the correct chemotherapy regimen, AC, also known as Adriamycin and Cytoxan. The nurse advised me that in three weeks, I would lose my hair. Well, that time came, and I allowed my husband to do the honors of shaving my head. Unfortunately, that ended with a trip to the barbershop.

I saw Dr. Vogel in November, and we went over my treatment plan. My final results indicated that I needed to start Herceptin, Taxotere, and Carboplatin. I started my second round of chemo treatment in November of 2005 and finished in March 2006.

March was a very busy month for us. I had to go to the Moffitt Center again for removal of two breast tumors and lymph nodes. The doctor at the Moffitt center advised me that I had an 85% chance the cancer would *not* return. I was relieved!

In June of 2006, I underwent thirty-three radiation treatments while still taking Herceptin. Fast-forward to March of 2007, after sixty-three doses of Herceptin, Dr. Vogel told me to have my port removed. This was such a happy day!

For some reason, I didn't schedule the port removal, and maybe that was a blessing in disguise. About two weeks later, I started to experience headaches. I thought it was a result of stressors since we were selling our house and dealing with a teenager ready to head off to college. As time progressed, the headaches persisted. I soon realized that I could not hold a pen to write, and I was occasionally falling in my own house as if I had one too many glasses of wine. I called Dr. Vogel, and he recommended that I have an MRI immediately.

I underwent the MRI and the radiologist came out with the films in her hand and told me, "Do not go home, go straight to Dr. Vogel's office. You have two tumors in your brain and massive swelling. The tumors measure 2.6 cm and 3 cm. One tumor is on the left temple side, and the other, on the back right side." I began to ask what the options for these types of tumors were. She said that Gamma Knife was the best choice. I drove directly to Dr. Vogel's office while my husband met me at the office. I was seen by the radiation oncologist and recommended the Gamma Knife procedure. The following week, the radiation was delivered.

After the procedure, Dr. Vogel put me on Tykerb, which was a brand-new drug at the time. The Tykerb kept the cancer at bay for a while.

In April of 2008, during a routine MRI scan, the radiologist unfortunately found a new 13 mm tumor in my brain. I underwent the Gamma Knife procedure yet again. Meanwhile, I was going on with my life, taking five chemo pills per day and feeling surprisingly well until the end of the year came; and once again, I found myself back for Gamma Knife. At this time, Dr. Vogel added Xeloda to my daily chemo regimen.

Throughout this journey, my family has been my rock. My husband and daughters stayed by my side during the good days and the bad days. My mother, Doe, has supported me the entire time. Whether it was flying down to visit me or just staying on the phone those extra minutes to let me know everything was going to be all right, she is always there for me. Other family and friends stepped up with love, prayers, and support. My sister, Tara, told me when my journey started to "pray, hope, and don't worry. Trust in Jesus's infinite mercy." I live by that saying to this day, and I am grateful to have such a wonderful sister by my side to help me with the crazy journey I call my survival journey.

I have been on chemotherapy drugs for over thirteen years. I am proud and blessed to say that I am cancer-free. My hair grew back thick and super curly; not what I was used to, but at least I have hair! It is with heartfelt thanks to Dr. Vogel and dedicated support staff that I am here today to tell my story of survival.

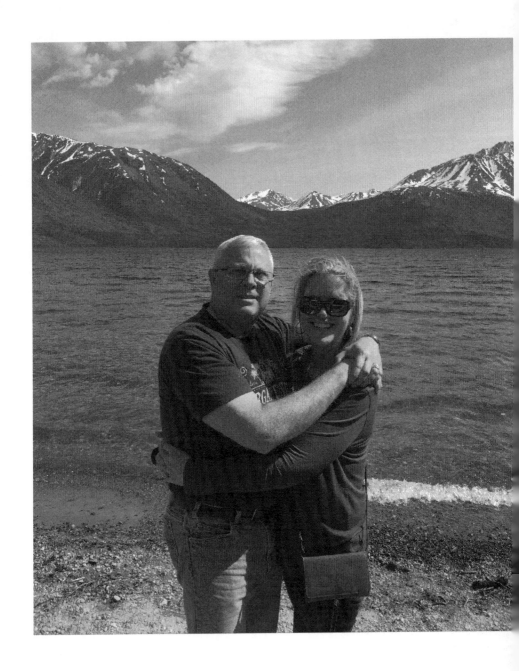

4: Karen

Karen's story is very abbreviated. She is a relative of mine, and, although she wanted her story told, I know few details of her clinical history.

Karen is of Ashkenazi Jewish heritage and was diagnosed at age twenty-eight in about 1985. Her mother was also diagnosed with breast cancer, but several years after Karen. She was tested and was BRCA negative

After mastectomy and appropriate adjuvant therapy, Karen developed systemic disease in 2003. She has been living with HER2 positive MBC for eighteen years, and like Kelly (chapter 8), lapatinib has been a mainstay of Karen's treatment for many years.

Unfortunately, Karen's clinical course was complicated by brain metastases requiring whole brain radiation therapy in 2006. As of June 2021, she continues treatment for MBC but is also significantly troubled by sequelae of her whole brain radiation.

Karen was diagnosed with breast cancer over thirty-five years ago, has had MBC for eighteen years, and has been living after a diagnosis of brain metastases for over fifteen years. She has been on lapatinib for twelve years.

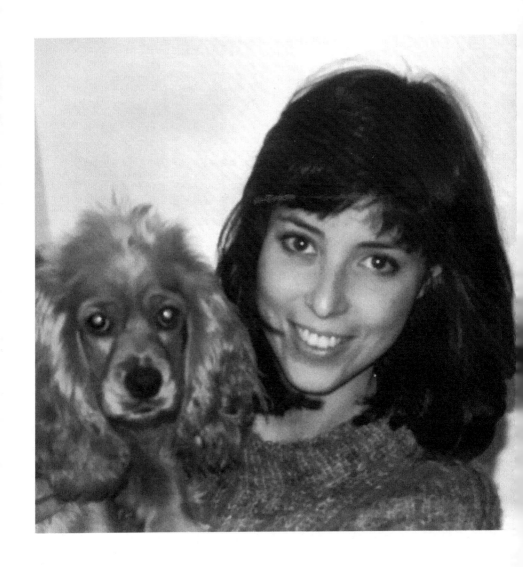

CHAPTER IX

Triple-Negative Breast Cancer

Introduction

Since the seminal paper by Perou's team subdividing breast cancer into intrinsic genetic subtypes (13, 14), triple-negative breast cancer has become the bad-girl subtype. Although constituting only 15% of breast cancer, it is highly aggressive, and survival statistics are worse than the other major subtypes which include luminal A (good risk estrogen-receptor positive), luminal B (poor risk estrogen receptor positive), and HER2 positive disease (which can be associated with either ER positive or ER negative subtypes).

While the intrinsic subtypes do recognize triple-negative breast cancer as an entity, it has proven to be heterogeneous and not uniformly associated with a poor prognosis. Investigators at Vanderbilt University have identified six distinct subgroups of TNBC, while others are working on further refining these subtypes (15, 16). One subtype (androgen receptor positive) seems to be associated with more indolent behavior.

Another encouraging observation about TNBC is the relatively reduced risk of late relapse after treatment for early stage (stages 1–3) disease. Currently, due to the effectiveness of adjuvant hormonal therapy in suppressing recurrences in ER positive disease, there are few relapses during endocrine adjuvant therapy. However, after five or ten years of adjuvant hormonal therapy, relapses can be seen fifteen, twenty, twenty-five, or even thirty years after initial diagnosis. Almost invariably, these late relapses are in patients with initially ER positive disease. Thus, a bright spot for TNBC is the relative rarity of relapses five years after initial diagnosis (48).

Several new drugs became available for the treatment of TNBC from 2019 to 2020. One such drug is atezolizumab (Tecentriq). This drug, in combination with nab-paclitaxel (Abraxane), became the first immunotherapeutic agent approved for use in MBC and specifically for TNBC (49). In patients who are PDL1 positive, response rates were superior for the combination as compared to Abraxane alone. Approximately 40% of the population in the clinical trial above were PDL1 positive by a specific assay and benefited significantly with the addition of this immunotherapeutic agent. Patients who were PDL1 negative did not benefit.

Two PARP inhibitors, olaparib and talazoparib, have shown significant activity in BRCA positive MBC. At least half of the patients in the clinical trials had TNBC. Thus if patients are both BRCA positive and have TNBC in the metastatic setting, this is another exciting therapeutic option (30).

Sacituzumab govitecan (IMMU-132; 50) is another new drug. It is a conjugated drug, meaning that it has multiple parts. One part is an antibody against TROP an anti-tumor target on tumor cells. Another part is *linked* to a *chemotherapeutic* agent. The TROP antibody acts as a Trojan horse bringing the chemotherapy directly into the tumor cells where the linker is cleaved, releasing the chemotherapy providing for more specific tumor cell kill. This drug was approved in April of 2020 and should provide an exciting new option for patients with triple-negative MBC.

Another immunotherapeutic agent, pembrolizumab (Keytruda), when added to chemotherapy, was found to be superior to chemotherapy alone, both in metastatic disease and in early stage TNBC (51, 52). It is the second immunotherapeutic compound approved for triple negative MBC by the FDA in combination with chemotherapy.

Thus, it should not be surprising that some patients with metastatic triple negative breast cancer defy the odds, and some may even behave indolently, hence the next few patients' histories.

1: Sue

In May of 1987, at age thirty, Sue was diagnosed with medullary carcinoma in the left breast. She underwent a lumpectomy and axillary dissection and was found to be node negative. CMF chemotherapy was given, and then she underwent radiation to the left breast.

She experienced a local recurrence in February 1989, which was noted to be ER and PR negative.

Sue received three cycles of Adriamycin and Cytoxan followed by Cytoxan, methotrexate, 5-fluorouracil, vincristine, and prednisone (CMFVP). She then was treated with two additional cycles of Adriamycin and Cytoxan.

Subsequently, she had multiple additional local recurrences. She was treated with local excision, photodynamic therapy, and ultimately, underwent a chest wall resection with extensive chest wall reconstruction in February 1993.

In December 2007, Sue opted for a prophylactic right mastectomy with the serendipitous finding of a 1.7 cm, grade 3, triple-negative invasive ductal carcinoma. She received Taxotere and carboplatin at that time.

In 2008, a lung lesion was removed, but it was an unrelated carcinoid tumor.

Sue has a strong family history for breast cancer and was tested for BRCA. She was found to have a mutation.

Sue is now 72 and has lived with breast cancer for 34 years, MBC for 32 years, and is 27 years since an extensive chest wall resection for multiple local relapses. Professionally, she works as a cancer patient advocate.

1, Sue: Takeaway

Sue, like 70% of BRCA1 carriers, had a TNBC. Similar to 40% of BRCA carriers, she also developed a subsequent cancer in the other breast many years after initial diagnosis.

The most striking part of Sue's story is the apparent cure of metastatic local disease, which was refractory to radiation therapy, chemotherapy, and photodynamic therapy, which was available in the 1990's as a treatment for breast cancer. Unfortunately, this control was only achieved after a deforming surgical chest wall resection, which included rib removal.

Although reconstructed with mesh and a skin graft, Sue's heart can be seen prominently beating beneath the thin skin graft and mesh.

Typically, multiple chest wall recurrences are ultimately associated with disseminated disease to vital organs. *However,* Sue's story and Beverly's, to follow, show that such dissemination is *not inevitable.*

Sue's Story

In 1987, at age forty, I was diagnosed with stage 2 medullary carcinoma, a type of breast cancer. It was estrogen negative and progesterone negative, and thirty-nine removed nodes were negative. All seemed very positive at that time.

However, soon after my diagnosis, we lost my 51-year-old sister to breast cancer. We mourned her loss and then came the possibility of losing my life. I was thrust into recovering from a lumpectomy, radiation, and chemotherapy. It was, to say the least, a very difficult time for my entire family. Having three children presented a variety of worries and thoughts. How could I assure them that I was going to be OK? How could I possibly help my sister's three daughters, as well as my brother and his children, cope? I remember how distraught my parents were and yet how tirelessly they were supporting me.

I quickly realized that I needed to find the right *team* of physicians to help me and to ultimately help my family as well. I chose to leave the care of my first oncologist because he made it clear that he wanted to be the sole decision maker with regard to my health care. Fortunately, I found the perfect breast cancer oncologist researcher to work *with* me and not for me. He has been a huge informational source and educator and assisted me in obtaining various opinions throughout six future recurrences. He also recommended that I join a new breast cancer support group. I did so and soon began to establish an educational arm for a nonprofit organization. Seminars began to surface. Speakers were invited from near and far to present information on breast cancer care to our community.

Then, I experienced a setback in 1989 when I recurred for the first time. I had never heard of a *skin recurrence*, and yet skin is the largest organ in the body. My oncologist suggested that I seek three opinions. I traveled from Georgetown University Medical Center to the University of Pennsylvania to MD Anderson Cancer Center in Texas—a one-week opinion tour.

When I arrived at Georgetown, I was introduced to a research oncologist. To make a long story short, I asked her not to give me statistics, just a recommendation for a treatment. However, within the first three minutes, she did just the opposite! She gave me a five-year survival opinion, after which I did not hear one more word. Now, I would have to ask the other physicians for their survival estimate so that I could have comparisons. I also made a very conscious decision to *prove* the Georgetown physician wrong! My mindset became clear to all. I am *not* a statistic!

Ultimately, decisions were made with regards to a mastectomy and an aggressive chemotherapy regimen. Timing became a positive for this untimely diagnosis. My oldest child was getting married and presented me with a wonderful diversion. I realized that I could handle several projects at once: surgery, treatment, wedding plans, and educational events. Keeping my calendar filled was my new mantra.

However, a month after my daughter's wedding, I again experienced a recurrence. This time, after consulting with several radiation oncologists, I chose to proceed with a research protocol involving *radiation hyperthermia*.

Once completed, three out of four lesions on the skin of my chest wall disappeared. The fourth was hoped to be scar tissue. I had to wait three months to have it biopsied, but unfortunately, my fourth recurrence was then detected.

Soon after, while participating at an event with physicians and researchers from around the country, I was introduced to a person from the NIH who discussed a research program called *photodynamic therapy*.

It was a difficult treatment, but I was optimistic that it would be effective against my chest wall recurrences. About two years later, it was recommended that a *PT*-treated area be biopsied to clear the way for a plastic surgical procedure. Unfortunately, the biopsy result was positive once again—recurrence number 5.

At about this same time, a very small Norwegian research study was presented to me by my medical oncologist. It involved a *chest wall resection*. Specifically, a large portion of the skin from my chest wall in the region of recurrence would be removed. I was fortunate to have been referred to a surgical oncologist who had performed a similar surgery in the past. He gave me the options of waiting to see what might present itself or to move forward with the surgery now. I was not an advocate of the watch-and-wait plan, so I moved forward with resection in early 1993. I was fortunate to have taken this course of action as more cancer was discovered at the time of the procedure. All went very well.

Meanwhile, genetic research presented me with the definitive answers. Although my oncologist and I assumed that I had a familial tendency for my cancer, there was no data to confirm this. However, within a few years, genetic research began to explode! I was diagnosed as BRCA1 positive, and seventeen family members probably share this mutation group. In addition, I also became a triple-negative breast cancer survivor.

In 2007, as a twenty-year survivor, I chose to undergo a contralateral prophylactic mastectomy. I wanted to have this performed in 1989. At that time, I was told that my insurance would not cover the cost. I soon realized that this was a lifesaving procedure when, once again, I was diagnosed with yet another recurrence.

Now, with a different type of carcinoma and with the knowledge of being a BRCA1 TNBC survivor decisions were made based on new information. It was mind boggling how many treatment advances existed since my last course of management. Even the side effect medications had improved!

Throughout the years, I worked for a large nonprofit cancer support program. I helped to establish educational programs as well as support groups, which I still continue to facilitate at medical facilities today. I feel blessed to have personally witnessed the remarkable research that has made some breast cancers a chronic illness, like diabetes. This is quite an improvement from many years prior.

As a long-term survivor, I have watched all my children settle into their professions, marry, and present me with the icing on the cake: eleven grandchildren! They always made me laugh, assisted me in the many programs that I was involved in, and most importantly, they have given me unconditional love and support.

My sister's three daughters are like my own. They are part of my cheering squad, and I appreciate their efforts, especially after losing their own mother. My oldest niece was the first to be tested for the BRCA gene after being diagnosed with breast cancer at thirty-four. Testing had just begun, and thankfully, she was able to reap the benefits of so many new discoveries. Today, she is a twenty-eight-year survivor!

My sister passed in 1987. However, each and every time I hear of new protocols, immunotherapy, new radiation therapy, diagnostics, and surgical breakthroughs, I believe that she and so many other breast cancer heroes have paved the way for all that has become available today and in the future. She once told me that I was going to be OK. Through it all, I believed her. It is now 2021, and I certainly proved that Georgetown physician wrong and my sister right!

I have been asked many times what the secret to my survivorship is. The answer is easy. Keep your calendar filled with the things you love and never say never!

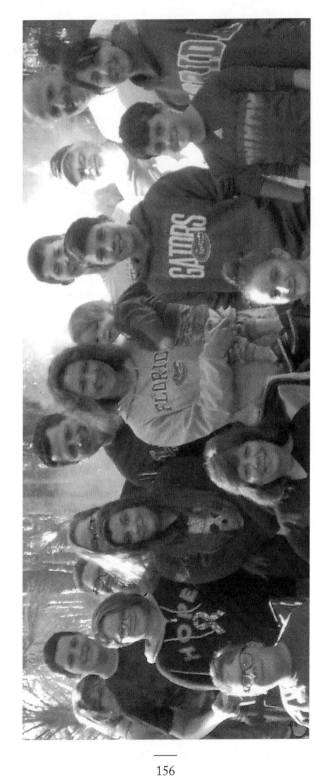

2: Beverly

Beverly underwent a right lumpectomy and sentinel node biopsy for a 3.5 cm triple-negative breast cancer with one positive lymph node in 2008 at the age of thirty-six.

Shortly after the lumpectomy, she underwent bilateral mastectomy with implant reconstruction. Her cancer was invasive carcinoma with lobular features. Dose-dense Adriamycin and Cytoxan was given and followed by dose-dense Taxol, which was changed to Abraxane. She underwent post mastectomy radiation.

In May 2010, Beverly underwent an MRI of the reconstructed breast, and a 1.1 cm recurrent lesion was identified within the radiated area of the right reconstructed breast. The tumor was removed. CMF chemotherapy was completed in November 2010.

Unfortunately, in February 2014, a skin punch biopsy of a small red area on the reconstructed breast returned as TNBC. It was excised in March 2014, but there was no further treatment

Beverly underwent bilateral breast reconstruction in May 2015. She is disease-free as of June 2021, seven years after two local recurrences of TNBC. Major takeaway points are summarized in Sue's take home messages. Just as in Sue's case, she had multiple local recurrences, but without spread to vital organs.

Beverly has had TNBC for eleven years and is now seven years disease free on no treatment after her last local relapse.

Beverly's Story: My Journey So Far

In 2008, my life changed forever with the diagnosis of breast cancer at the age of thirty-six. I had been undergoing mammograms since 2000 because I palpated a lump. At that time, a biopsy was negative for breast cancer. In 2008, I was late for my annual mammogram because I broke my left humerus and could not lift my arm. I noticed my nipple was itchy and had a discharge. I then performed a breast exam and found a lump.

I scheduled a mammogram and required an ultrasound. I was recommended to proceed with an MRI and was subsequently notified that I likely had breast cancer. I was at work when I got the call. I called my husband, and he said, "Don't worry, we will get through this." At home, we hugged and cried. My son walked in from school and said, "Get a room" (not knowing what was going on). We all laughed. Laughter truly is the best medicine! We then told our son and twin girls after dinner that night. It was one of the hardest things I've ever had to do in my life. I was scheduled to undergo a biopsy and was diagnosed with triple-negative breast cancer. I proceeded with bilateral mastectomy and reconstruction. A week later, I began chemotherapy. Chemo was long, painful, and exhausting, but I knew I had to fight to stay here for my family. I looked forward to getting on with my life!

After chemotherapy was complete, I underwent daily radiation for six weeks. Subsequently, I proceeded to finish my reconstruction. I could finally see a light at the end of this long tunnel. Then, in 2010, my breast started to itch again. I knew that my cancer had returned. My doctor did not believe me! My chiropractor recommended Dr. Vogel, and I rushed to see him. What a Godsend. I had workup with an MRI and then underwent resection of the recurrent breast cancer. I started chemo for the second time. It was another difficult road, but I had my husband, kids, family, and close friends by my side.

During this time, I found out that I was going to be a grandmother. Yay! This was something to look forward to. After I completed chemo, life was *great*. Unfortunately, in 2014, my breast started itching and I discovered another lump. My breast cancer always returned in the same spot. I had a biopsy that confirmed the cancer recurrence. I decided that I did not want more chemotherapy. I proceeded with surgical resection. There was more cancer discovered behind my implant, and I had the implant removed. In 2015, I went forward with reconstruction with a tram flap. It became infected, and I had to undergo more surgery. I now look like a science experiment gone wrong, but I don't care. I have my life, my family, and my close friends. That is all that matters. I am a grandmother to five beautiful granddaughters. The most important thing is to stay positive and believe in miracles. God has walked with me every step of the way. My story is far from over.

3: Margaret Lynn

In June 2011, at age forty-nine, Margaret Lynn was diagnosed with a left breast cancer. It was invasive ductal carcinoma, triple negative, and grade 3.

She underwent neoadjuvant Taxotere, Adriamycin, and Cytoxan for six cycles.

In December 2011, she underwent a left lumpectomy. At that time, a 1.2 cm residual tumor with negative sentinel nodes was found. However, postoperatively, she opted for a complete mastectomy. While no additional tumor was found in the breast, four additional lymph nodes were involved with cancer.

Margaret Lynn did well until September 2013 when a tumor was discovered in the left lung. It was removed and found to be a 1.5 cm TNBC. The tumor was 25% positive for androgen receptors.

FoundationOne next-generation genomic sequencing identified KRAS amplification RETT636M, TP53Y327, and CUL3K610, but no targetable mutations.

No antineoplastic therapy was given in the stage IV NED situation.

Margaret Lynn is now eight years after surgical removal of the lung metastasis and remains disease-free on no therapy.

3, Margaret Lynn: Takeaway

In contrast to the prior two patients, both of whom had extraordinary clinical courses after multiple local recurrences of TNBC, Margaret Lynn experienced a lung recurrence.

It is hard to know how applicable Margaret's situation is to others with oligometastatic (single site) recurrence of TNBC. I do have one other patient who underwent resection for oligometastatic lung metastasis with prolonged disease-free survival. Neither Margaret Lynn nor this other patient received chemotherapy after lung resection.

Given the unrelenting quest for effective therapies against TNBC, consider these anecdotal cases illustrating potential effectiveness of local therapy for oligometastatic disease. Additionally, focal aggressive radiation therapy such as stereotactic body radiation therapy (SBRT) could be an option for some oligometastatic patients.

Margaret Lynn's Story

My name is Lynn. Legally it's Margaret Lynn, and in April of 2011, I was a happily married mom to five children. I was many years into a career in my county emergency management department and was looking forward to my fiftieth birthday upcoming. My primary doctor suggested that I have a mammogram. I told him they were not effective for me because I had dense breast disease. He explained that mammograms had improved and recommended that I proceed. I went for the exam, and basically forgot about it until I received the phone call. I was on my balcony at a luxury hotel in Fort Lauderdale for the Governor's Hurricane Conference when I was told my mammogram needed follow-up. It was my daughter's nineteenth birthday. And so, my journey with cancer began.

I was diagnosed with stage 2 triple-negative breast cancer. I suggested removal of breasts but was told it wasn't necessary. I was not told that triple-negative disease was a very aggressive form of cancer with a good chance of coming back. If I had been given this information, I would have insisted on removal. I was only told that it was not a hormone-driven cancer. Therefore, I would not have to complete my partial hysterectomy. So, I thought I was winning. I went through six months of chemotherapy, with Neulasta shots after each round to help my blood counts. I lost weight, as the chemo diet is pretty effective. However, I do not recommend this as the way to lose weight. I was diagnosed with two tumors in my left breast. One was necrotic and the other was on my nerves. I named them after my exes. I thought it was apropos. The chemotherapy shrank the tumors so much that guide wires were necessary, and the procedure removed less of my breast. Three weeks later, I proceeded with radiation planning. I noticed that with minimal manipulation there was discomfort. I called my surgeon from the parking lot and was told to come in the next day.

While I lay on my side for the ultrasound, I asked what we were looking for. "Black holes," she said. "Like that one?" I asked, as I pointed to a quarter-size shape. She left the room to get biopsy equipment. When she came back, I said that my axillary area under my arm hurt. She assured me it was in the tail of my breast. I said, "Tell that to my arm pit, it hurts." So to humor me, she examined my axilla where two additional tumors were noted. This seemed to be three tumors in three weeks! I don't have that many exes, so being an election year, I named them after presidential candidates. I think naming the tumors gave me a sense of control in a situation where I felt as though I had no control. Biopsy of all three lesions showed cancer. I was asked if I objected to having my breast removed. I said take to them both. Once again, I was told that it was not necessary. This time, I insisted. I did not want to worry about every little twinge in my healthy breast. Besides, I asked, "You gonna make me a saggy one to match?" So on the day after Valentine's Day, the girls were gone. In my defense, they tried to kill me!

Before a mastectomy, you see a plastic surgeon to discuss your options regarding reconstruction. If you decide on implants, expanders are placed at the time of the mastectomy. The plastic surgeon I saw had *no* sense of humor, something I depend on to cope with difficult situations. I had expectations of gravity-defying tatas, with cleavage and pink nipples. I was told that I would likely be a B cup without cleavage or nipples. They tattoo them after you heal! Having never had a tattoo, I didn't want my first one to be a nipple and expressed my disappointment by asking if I could get a tattoo of two turtles facing each other. That way, my husband could make them kiss. I was told that I would have to go to a tattoo parlor for that, and just where did I expect them to find pink nipples? "From a dead redhead," I told him. No humor. Zilch. I thanked him for his time and passed on reconstruction. Reconstruction is a personal decision, and I did what was best for me. Perhaps never having much in the breast department to begin with made this decision easier. I know that being married for many years was a factor as well. As I could not have any of the things I desired, and the hubby and I could carry on without them, I did not see the point of going through all that at my age. So now, I'm aerodynamically styled!

Unfortunately, the cancer returned. It spread to my lung, and I was a stage 4. As there is no stage 5, I went alone to make my funeral arrangements. I paid for them in full. I did not want my husband or daughters to have to deal with it. I lost faith in my team for all the things they didn't tell me, so I changed to University of Miami's Miller School of Medicine where I met (and fell a little in love with) Dr. Charles Vogel. He is the one I credit with saving my life. He is a lovely man and will tell you it's a team effort, and it is!

I'm part of that team too. All teams need a captain, and I was blessed the day he became my doctor.

The robotic-assisted surgery to remove my lung tumor involved only one overnight stay and seems to have done the trick. I am now eight years cancer-free!

That is the summary of my cancer journey. It does not include all the fear, tears, financial struggles, pain, and plain misery that accompanied my days. Neither does it include the moments of joy, pure happiness, and deeper bonding as family and friends. May you be as pleasantly surprised as I was by the people who show up for you on your journey.

A friend who knows me and my pride well told me to just say thank you when offered help. Take the help being offered to you! It may be all they can do to show you love, so let them. Don't deny someone a blessing. We all need as many as we can get.

CHAPTER X

Judy Ann: A Miracle of Science

At age thirty-eight, in 2003, Judy was diagnosed with ductal carcinoma in situ. She underwent left mastectomy. No invasive cancer was found, and she received no adjuvant systemic therapy or radiation.

Judy relapsed in August 2013 with invasive cancer that was ER positive, PR positive and negative for HER2. PET-CT showed numerous involved lymph nodes including bilateral supraclavicular and axillary, left paratracheal, and mediastinal nodes in addition to disease in the left chest wall parasternal soft tissues and sternum. She received Abraxane chemotherapy with good response seen on PET-CT in December 2013.

In February 2014, enlarging nodal disease was noted on exam. However, CT scan showed that most of the disease had responded except for a left anterior-superior mediastinal chest wall mass that was invading the anterior chest and sternum.

By March 2014, Judy Ann had progressive disease by PET scan and began Arimidex until June 2014, when she discontinued it in preparation for the PALOMA-3 trial. Unfortunately, it closed before she could enroll. This would have given her an option to receive palbociclib, then investigational.

Faslodex started in July 2014, and she restarted anastrozole with it. She developed progressive disease in September 2014.

She began Xeloda in September 2014, and Navelbine was added in October 2014, due to poor response with Xeloda alone.

At relapse, Taxotere, Adriamycin, and Cytoxan were started in November 2014. After only two doses, clinical progression occurred with significant worsening of her pain.

A FoundationOne report indicated FGFR positivity, and she began Lucitanib on clinical trial in January 2015. The left chest wall mass was biopsied in January 2015, revealing invasive ductal carcinoma, ER positive, PR negative, and HER2 negative. Dose reductions were needed due to thyroid function abnormalities and low platelets. At the lower dose, she again progressed. Judy Ann went back on a higher dose and her last dose of Lucitanib was in July 2015. This investigational drug was subsequently found to be ineffective in breast cancer.

In September 2015, Judy was seen at the National Cancer Institute to assess eligibility for an investigational tumor infiltrating lymphocytes (TIL) clinical trial. Please read Judy's story for a miracle of science.

Judy Ann's Story

Five years ago, I was dying with only a few months to live. My breast cancer had returned, and the fight was almost over. I spent as much time with my friends and family as I could. I had no more bucket-list plans, and I intended to curl up with my cats and read books or watch TV until I died.

But I had one last chance at the brass ring. And I took it.

When I was diagnosed in 2013, it was a heavy blow. Metastatic (or stage 4) breast cancer is "treatable but not curable." For obvious reasons, I was suddenly very motivated to learn everything I could about my disease. My cousin, a patient advocate for many years, advised me to go to a comprehensive cancer center and to try to get into clinical trials.

Two years later, more than a dozen treatments had failed me. I had been treated by Dr. Charles Vogel at the University of Miami, and we had tried various types of hormonal therapy and chemotherapy. I had even been in a clinical trial for a drug called Lucitanib, an FGFR1 inhibitor, which had some magic and bought me almost six months. At first, my tumors seemed to disappear, and both Dr. Vogel and I were excited by the results. But I experienced a host of side effects and practically had Dr. Vogel on speed dial. We were able to manage problems with blood pressure and thyroid function, but ultimately, my platelet count got too low. We had to reduce the dosage until that too failed.

That's when I met a researcher at the National Cancer Institute. At an advocacy training called Project LEAD, she told me about their clinical trial. More importantly, she told me that it might work.

Dr. Vogel's team quickly pulled my records together so that I could apply for the trial. A few weeks later, I arrived for duty at the National Institutes of Health in Bethesda, Maryland. The trial was for immunotherapy using tumor infiltrating lymphocytes (TIL for short). Here is how it works: Inside my tumors were T-cells, which were able to recognize my cancer. But the cancer was able to trick these T-cells into thinking it wasn't a threat; thus, the cancer avoided setting off the alarm and kept my T-cells from multiplying and attacking. The team at the NCI has created a treatment that is often able to overcome this resistance.

To be a candidate for this trial, you have to have at least two tumors. One that can be resected (to obtain the TIL), and one that they can watch to see if the treatment is working. With breast cancer patients, we often have bone-only disease. By the time we have tumors that can be surgically removed, the cancer has spread to the liver or lungs, and we are becoming too sick to endure the treatment. Some patients have brain metastases, and they also don't qualify for the trial. Because of these problems, I was the first breast cancer patient that was treated.

I was a good candidate because I had an easily accessible tumor in my right breast, and I was still fairly healthy. In August of 2015, my tumor was removed. They isolated the T-cells from my tumor. They fed them bits of my tumor to identify the cells that would attack my tumor. They then expanded these cells and filled an IV bag with 81 billion of them.

Unfortunately, it took four months to complete the work in the lab. Between my surgery (in August) and when my cells were ready (in December), I had really started to go down the rabbit hole. I was in a lot of pain. Tumors had spread throughout my liver. I understood that the odds of this treatment working were about 15% (not good), and I was doing my best to prepare myself for the unhappy but likely outcome.

I limped into the clinic at the NIH in December of 2015 and was there for almost a month. Prior to receiving my cells, I received high-dose chemotherapy to temporarily knock out my immune system. The post-treatment is grueling. Suffice it to say that, when I was finished, I felt battered and weak.

Despite the fact that I felt miserable, even before I left the clinic, I had a glimmer of hope. I knew that my tumors were shrinking. They continued to shrink, and I stopped taking my pain meds cold turkey. A few weeks later, my energy returned. By April, I was backpacking again on the Appalachian Trail. In May of 2016, I had my first clean scan. My cancer was gone, and it has stayed that way ever since.

Since news of my clinical trial was published, there's been a lot of excitement about the treatment I received. But my friend, received the same treatment—and it didn't work for her. To my knowledge, it hasn't worked for anyone else with breast cancer. Cindy was also a patient of Dr. Vogel's, and we all hoped she would have the same response that I did. Sadly, she joined the ranks of the forty-two thousand people who die of breast cancer each year and passed away just a few months after her treatment.

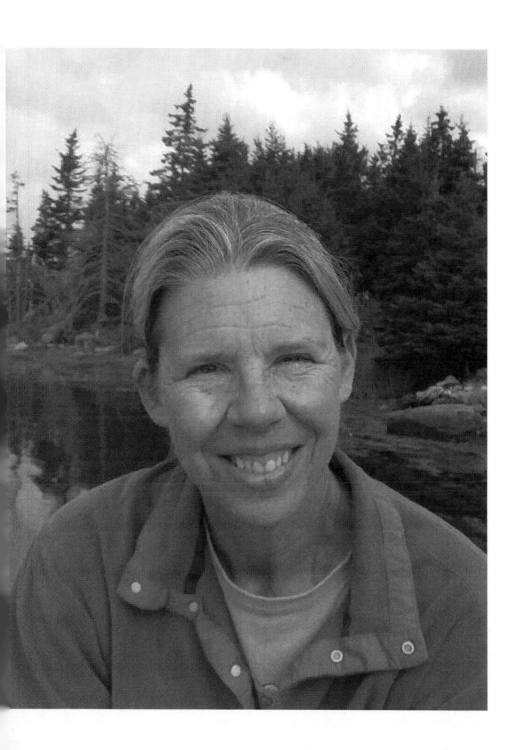

CHAPTER XI

Rebecca: A Miracle of Faith

Rebecca is from the Bahamas. In about 1986, at age 30, she was diagnosed with a five cm invasive ductal carcinoma which was, ER and PR negative. HER2 was not performed at that time.

She underwent a right lumpectomy followed by Cytoxan, Adriamycin, and 5-fluorouracil (CAF) for six doses.

Rebecca recurred within the right breast in 1992. She was treated with mastectomy after chemotherapy with CAF ×3, followed by Ifosfamide, VP-16, and Carboplatin. No reconstruction was performed.

Unfortunately, in 1993, Rebecca developed an inflammatory-like recurrence on the right chest wall with additional tumor nodules on the surface of the left breast. Treatment with additional chemotherapy consisting of Mitomycin and Vinblastine helped the inflammatory changes, but after a couple of months of treatment, she chose to discontinue therapy and return to the Bahamas. She was only seen one additional time about six weeks after she went to the Bahamas. Although the tumor nodules on the left breast did not improve, she declined any further therapy.

Surprisingly, after 28 years in 2011, Rebecca reached out for advice.

She was not having a breast cancer issue, but rather heart failure. The latter was almost certainly due to Adriamycin chemotherapy years earlier.

Metastatic workup revealed no evidence of cancer. She adamantly denied receiving any form of treatment for the breast cancer, including alternative therapy or local Bahamian remedies.

Recognizing that her situation regarding metastatic breast cancer was rare and highly unusual, she was asked again what helped her cancer. Her answer was "My *faith* and *prayer.*"

Rebecca: Takeaway

Spontaneous Cure of MBC

Going back to the seminal paper by Greenberg et al. (1), it is recalled that of 1,500 patients treated with CAF chemotherapy for MBC, only 2.5% were disease-free at fifteen years. These data and others have led physicians to consider MBC as "essentially incurable." As the reader has seen, "incurable" does not mean untreatable; and many patients can live long, productive, and relatively comfortable lives for many years. Further, these authors feel that there are some patients, especially with HER2-positive MBC who are cured. Many such patients in long-term remission are afraid of stopping Herceptin knowing that MBC is incurable. However, women like Andrea (chapter 7) stopped Herceptin after eight years of remission and remain disease-free thirteen years later. There are other reports of spontaneous remissions/cures of breast cancer that have appeared in the literature (53) to which we now add Rebecca's story.

Rebecca's Story: My Journey with Metastatic Breast Cancer

My name is Rebecca. I am the youngest of nine children (twins). I am married, and together we have two adult children, one daughter-in-law, and one grandson. I would like to share with you my journey with metastatic breast cancer.

In June of 1986, while performing a self-breast examination, I discovered a lump in my breast. One week later, I went to the gynecologist. In addition to the lump, I was two months' pregnant. After examining me, I was told that the lump may be related to my pregnancy. I was not alarmed because I knew that pregnancy causes certain changes in your body. The lump developed with time, and after my daughter was born in January of 1987, it persisted. During my postnatal checkup, I expressed my concern to the physician, who then referred me to an oncologist. A mammogram was performed, as well as a biopsy. By the time I recovered, my husband already knew the results. The doctor asked to see us both the following morning.

By the expression on my husband's face, I knew something was terribly wrong. I was informed that I had breast cancer and a mastectomy was recommended in order to prolong my life. The shock of it did not hit me until we were on our way home. I thought that I had just awakened from a bad dream. All kinds of negative thoughts went through my mind. I said to myself, *God what have I done? Here I am, a young wife—married just five years—and mother of a four-year-old and six-week-old baby. How can I die now?* My journey with the Lord began that very moment. You see, I was raised in the Episcopal faith, but I did not know Christ as my personal Savior.

When we arrived home, we broke the news to my mother, who was visiting at the time. She was bewildered, as I had an older sister who died of cancer ten years prior. We watched as she suffered helplessly. In my mother's mind, she could not believe that she would be experiencing this again. We sought a second opinion from another oncologist. I was given two options: mastectomy or lumpectomy. I decided on the latter, with the removal of the lymph nodes, chemotherapy, and radiation. The operation was performed, and it was discovered that the cancer had only spread to two of the lymph nodes. I was thankful to God for this, as the lump had been present for a long time, and cancer could have spread throughout my entire body. This is what the power of prayer can do when you trust God. Sometimes it seems as though God is a million miles away, but he is not. He reminds us that he "will never leave us or forsake us" (Hebrews 13:5).

Five years after my diagnosis, I noticed a swelling in the same breast. I waited almost two weeks before seeking medical attention. A mammogram was performed, and I was assured that everything was all right. I was given antibiotics to treat a presumed infection. The antibiotics did not work. I returned to the doctor's office for further testing. Again, I prayed and asked God to give me the strength and courage that whatever the results of the biopsy, whether good or bad, I would be able to cope with the situation. Two days later, I was told that the cancer had recurred and that I would require a series of tests, chemotherapy, and a mastectomy. God is good, because again all tests showed that the cancer had not spread to other parts of my body. Because I had claimed my healing, the devil tried to show me negative signs to make me doubt. In spite of this, I thank God for the positive-thinking people he had placed in my life, along with the support from my husband, mother, and siblings. Negative thinkers and doubters can cause you to fall short of what God has for you. Again, trust and faith played a big part in my prognosis.

When the cancer returned a third time, I had four lumps on the other side. This time, I received intense chemotherapy requiring hospitalization for three days at a time. After undergoing treatment for several months, I informed my oncologist that I was not going to undergo any more chemotherapy. It did not appear as though it was effective in dispelling the cancer. Besides, I had faith in God. He agreed and recommended testing after Christmas. As it was a few weeks before Christmas, I guess he did not want to spoil the holidays in case the tests came back concerning. Thankfully, before Christmas, three of the lumps disappeared.

One lump remained and became quite large over time. This was a test of my faith. Each time the doctor decided to remove it, he changed his mind. All this time, I continued to speak to my mountain. It was the night after Christmas—a year later—I said to God, "You know, Lord, it would be the greatest gift if you would just take this lump away." When I looked down, I noticed that the skin around the lump was wrinkled. This was a sign that the lump was shrinking. I quickly showed it to my husband, who also noticed the same thing. By January, the lump was completely gone. My doctor was totally amazed and wanted to know what I had done. He said that he had never seen anything like that before. He threw his hand in the air and said he took no credit for it. He inquired about my diet. I told him that it was through prayer and fasting that I was healed. He asked me to remember two of his terminally ill patients in prayer.

In 2011, I became tired easily, especially when I walked up a hill. I expressed my concern to the doctor and was referred to a cardiologist. It was discovered that my heart was only working at 20%. He informed me that the chemotherapy destroyed the left ventricle of my heart. I was advised to have a checkup with my oncologist, as I had not visited the oncologist in eighteen years. After an online search, I discovered that Dr. Charles Vogel was still practicing. He was very happy to see me. When I told him about my heart condition, he said that one of the drugs that I was treated with caused heart failure.

I continue follow-up visits with Dr. Vogel, and it has been another eight years. He always states that I am truly a miracle and that in all his years of practicing that he has never seen anything like this. God not only gives us promises, a dream, or his love. He gives us all kinds of tools, resources, and guides—such as medical professionals—to help us fulfill our trust in him.

Since 1987, my spiritual eyes have been opened and prayer and fasting have become a part of my life. Reading God's Word, meditating on his promises, and doing his will are very important to me. My journey was a long one, not knowing whether I was going to live to see my children become adults and also witness my grandson grow up. I am blessed that my son is now thirty-seven years old and employed with the federal government as an auditor. My daughter is now thirty-three years old and is a researcher for one of the Bahamas' leading psychiatrists. I am still gainfully employed and look forward to retiring next year to spend more time with my family.

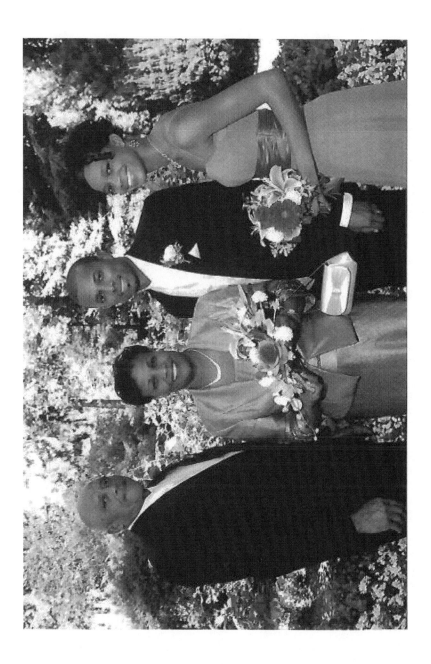

CHAPTER XII

Postscript

As stated in Judy's story on page 164, when diagnosed with MBC, her doctor told her it was "treatable but not curable." All too often, many patients only hear the words not curable, and all subsequent discussion becomes a blur. This is a statement repeated daily by oncologists to patients around the world, bringing with it an outpouring of emotions, including sadness, dread, fear, and helplessness.

This book was written to show that long and productive lives after a diagnosis of MBC is possible. While the patients chosen here are examples, we could have chosen hundreds of others from within our practice over the past couple of decades with similarly long periods of disease control. Likewise, every oncologist has many such patients in their practice. These authors also feel that even though we speak of incurability, certain patients may have been cured of MBC, especially some within the HER2 positive disease subset.

In this computer age, many patients read about MBC and the statistics. Hopefully, this book and the patients' own stories will help the MBC reader believe this: "*I am not a statistic.*"

CHAPTER XIII

Acknowledgments

The authors would, first and foremost, like to thank all of our patients, including those within the pages of this book. They have taught us, as physicians, lessons in strength, courage, compassion, empathy, and humility as, together, we battle a relentless and ever-changing disease process.

We especially thank Maricela Espino, who helped organize and type every element of this book.

We acknowledge the contributions of many grateful patients who donated to the Sylvester Comprehensive Cancer Center, University of Miami Miller School of Medicine (Deerfield Beach) Research Fund, which, in part, funded Mrs. Espino's efforts.

The authors would also like to thank the Marketing and Communications team at Baptist Health and UHealth–University of Miami Health System for granting permission to reprint their photos of Drs. Vogel and Freedman, respectively.

While the patient and their oncologist are the core team in this critical fight against a constantly mutating adversary, it truly does take a village to treat each metastatic breast cancer patient. The primary medical team including the medical oncologist, surgical oncologist and radiation oncologist also includes nurse practitioners; nurse navigators; chemotherapy nurses; physician assistants; intake and scheduling personnel; diagnostic and interventional radiologists; nutritionists; psychologists/psychiatrists;

genetic counselors; lymphedema specialists; radiation therapists; medical assistants; social workers; financial counselors; pharmacists; and others who all work together in support of common goals! All team members work to help extend life and maximize quality of life while maintaining the dignity of the individual under their collective care.

Some of the warm, caring medical professionals who have helped us care for patients in this book and others like them over several decades are Colleen Brennan-Doran, RN; Shirley Godbold, RN; Karen Hernandez, PA; Kerry Ritchey, ARNP; Cynthia Frankel, RN; Dawn East, RN; and Catriona Byrne, RN.

Chapter XIV

Biosketch

Charles L. Vogel, MD, FACP

Born in Rockaway Beach, New York, Dr. Charles L. Vogel was educated at Princeton, Yale Medical School, Emory University, and the US National Cancer Institute (NCI). From 1969 to 1973, he established a Solid Tumor Research Institute in Uganda for the NCI. Returning to the United States, he established the first oncology ward at an inner-city hospital, Grady Memorial, in Atlanta, Georgia. He started his specialization in breast cancer in 1975 as chief of the division of breast cancer at the Comprehensive Cancer Center, University of Miami, Florida. Over the next four decades, he was a pioneer in establishing cancer clinical trials in the community setting. He was one of the key clinical research contributors to the Herceptin development program, and another manuscript changed the prescribing guidelines worldwide for Neulasta to prevent chemotherapy-induced infection. Since January 2021, he relocated his practice of breast medical oncology to the Miami Cancer Institute (Plantation, Florida) of Baptist Health South.

CHAPTER XV

Biosketch

Laura M. Freedman, MD

D r. Freedman is a radiation oncologist with more than two decades of experience. Born in Detroit, Michigan, she was educated at the University of Michigan Medical School and completed residency training at MD Anderson Cancer Center in Houston, Texas. She began her career at Wayne State University and the Karmanos Cancer Institute. She joined faculty at the University of Michigan before joining Sylvester Comprehensive Cancer Center in 2011. Over the past twenty years, she has published articles focused on education and has been involved in multiple national committees for the field of radiation oncology. She is currently a board examiner for the American Board of Radiology. Her practice includes breast cancer and lung cancer, as well as head and neck cancers, and she is actively involved in the community with participation in numerous outreach events. She is currently the director of radiation oncology at the Deerfield Beach location and an associate professor of the University of Miami Miller School of Medicine. She lives in Parkland, Florida, and enjoys travel, exercise, and spending time with her husband, Jeff, sons Scott, Zach, and Matthew, and two dogs, Lucy and Oreo.

References

1. Greenberg et al. J. Clinic Onc 14:2197–2205, 2016
2. Siegel et al. Ca: A Cancer Journal for Clinicians 70: 7–30, 2020
3. Narod S. Jama Oncology 1:888–896, 2015
4. Van Maaren et al. Eur J Cancer 101:134–142, 2018
5. Carey et al. Jama 285:363–385, 2019
6. Jemal A. et al. J. Clinical Oncology 36:14–24, 2018
7. Kimberly D. Ca: A Cancer Journal for Clinicians 69:363–385, 2019
8. Vogel et al. Cancer 70:129–135, 1992
9. Zeichner et al. Breast Cancer Basic and Clin. Res. 9:1–9, 2015
10. Giordano et al. Cancer 100:44–52, 2004
11. Zeichner et al. Breast Ca Res Treat 153:617–624, 2015
12. Schneider J. G., Khalil D. N. Breast Cancer Res Treat. 134:1125–32, 2012
13. Sorlie T. et al. Proc Nat'l Acad Sci USA 98: 10869–10874, 2001
14. Perou C. M. et al. Nature 406:747–52, 2000
15. Lehmann B. D. et al. J. Clin Invest 121:2750–67, 2011
16. Ahn S. G. et al. J. Breast Cancer 19:223–230, 2016
17. Aebi et al. Lancet Oncology 15:156–163, 2014
18. Rivera et al. The Breast Journal 8:2–9, 2002
19. Willner J., Kiricuta I. C., et al. Int. J. Radiation Oncology Biol Phys 37:853–863, 1997
20. Chand A. R., Ziauddin, et al. Clinical Breast Cancer 17:326–35, 2017
21. Lambertini M. Lancet Oncology 20:471–472, 2020
22. Ganon Y. and Tetu A. B. Cancer 64:892–898, 1989
23. Vogel: Clinical Breast Cancer 14:1–9, 2014

24. Mahtani R., Stein A., et al. Clinical Therapeutics 31:1-2371–2378, 2009
25. Ellis M. J.: Jama; 302 774–780, 2009
26. Raphael J., Lefebvre C., et al. Target Oncology 15: 723–32, 2020
27. Howell A. et al. Ann. Oncol. 3:611–617, 1992
28. Wolpert N., Warner E., et al. Clin Breast Ca 1:57–63, 2000
29. Ottini L., Rizzolo P., et al. Breast Cancer Res Treat 116:577–86, 2009
30. Mohyuddin BMC Cancer 20:507–516, 2020
31. Arciero C. A., Guo Y., et al. Clinical Breast Cancer 19:236–245, 2019
32. Gianni L., Pienkowski T., et al. Lancet Oncology 13:25–32, 2012
33. Swain et al. New Eng J. Med 372:724–734, 2015
34. Schettini F., Pascual, et al. Cancer Treat Rev. Mar; 84:101965, 2020
35. Blackwell et al. J. Clin Oncol 28:1124–1130, 2010
36. Mahtani et al. J. Clin Oncol 19:5823–5824, 2020
37. Brufsky A. M. et al. Clin Cancer Res. 17:4834–4843, 2011
38. Hurvitz S. A., et al. Clin Cancer Res. 25:2433–2441, 2019
39. Ramakrishna N. et al. J Clin Oncol. 36:2804–2807, 2018
40. Freedman R. A., et al. J Clin Oncol. 38:1081–189, 2019
41. Saura C. et al. J Clin Oncol. Volume 38, issue 27, 3138–3149, 2020
42. Lin N., Murthy R. K., et al. N. Eng J Med. 382:597–609, 2020
43. Lin J. U. et al. ASCO abstract 1005, 2020
44. Brown et al., Lancet Oncol. August; 18:1049–1060, 2017
45. Brown et al., Neuro-Oncology 15:1429–1437, 2013
46. Brown et al., J Clin Oncol. 38:1019–1029, 2020
47. Perez E. A., Suman V. J., et al. J. Clin Oncol 29:4491–4497, 2011
48. Reddy S. M., Barcenas C. H., et al. Brit J Ca 118:17–23, 2017
49. Schmid et al. New Eng J. Med 379:2108–2121, 2018
50. Bardia et al. New Eng J. Med 380:741–751, 2019
51. Cortes et al. J. Clin Oncol 38 (issue 15) suppl.
52. Schmid et al. New Eng J. Med 382:810–821, 2020
53. Jessey: J Nat Sci Biol Med 2:43–49, 2011

INDEX

G

Gamma Knife, 129, 137, 142, 144–45
Gemzar, 54, 68, 85
genes, 6, 8, 17, 19, 92, 108, 127
geneticist, 125
Georgia, 111–12, 122, 177
Georjean, 79–80
Gloria, 34–36, 43–44, 93
gynecologist, 38–39, 49, 55–56, 117, 169

H

hair, losing, 12, 36, 51–52, 57–58, 97, 124–25, 134–35, 140, 144–45
Henrietta, 17
HER2, 92
HER2 negative, 28, 38, 45, 57, 67, 73, 80, 107
HER2/neu, 6, 24, 50
HER2 positive, 35, 45, 97, 107, 116, 127, 129, 131, 134
Herceptin, 6–7, 24, 29–31, 35–36, 44, 92, 94, 96–97, 100–106, 111, 116–17, 119, 122–23, 125–28, 131–32, 134, 137, 144, 169
heterogeneity, 132
hormonal therapy, 17, 47–48, 55, 60–61, 77, 79, 85–86, 102–3, 107, 149, 164
Howell, Tony, 60

I

Ibrance, 42, 46, 54, 59, 64, 67, 73, 83, 85
immune system, 88–89, 165
immunotherapeutic agent, 150
immunotherapy, 5
infection, 12, 19, 86, 170
inhibitors, 5, 7, 46, 164
   aromatase, 44, 46, 55, 61, 80

J

Janice, 100–101
Jean, 123, 125, 127
Joan, 9–13
Joanne, 76–77, 80
Judith, 67–69
Judy Ann, 163–64

K

Kadcyla, 7, 94, 100, 104, 106, 123, 126, 137
Karen, 105, 143, 147
Kaye, 10, 18–19
Kelly, 96, 105, 122, 142–43, 147
Kirsten, 137–38
Krukenberg Tumor, 34
kyphoplasty, 94

L

lapatinib, 7, 94–95, 143, 147
Laura, 32
lesions, 47, 79, 101, 106, 137, 153, 161
letrozole, 12, 38, 46, 54–55, 59, 64, 67, 76–77, 79, 83–85, 96, 100, 102, 106
Lisa, 131–33
liver, 4, 6, 22, 32, 42, 77, 79, 85, 96, 100, 106, 108, 122, 132, 134, 137, 139, 165
liver lesions, 100–101, 106, 131
Lorraine, 83, 101–3
Lucitanib, 164
luminal A, 6–7, 45, 93, 149
luminal B, 6, 11, 45, 149
lump, 19, 35, 49, 68, 86, 117–18, 133, 143, 157–58, 169–71
lumpectomy, 4–5, 28, 35, 42, 73, 80, 94, 97, 104, 123, 139, 143, 151–52, 157, 170

lungs, 4, 6, 20, 22, 32, 84, 86–87, 90, 132, 134, 161, 165

Lupron, 45, 64, 76

lymphedema, 5, 38–39, 119

lymph nodes, 4–5, 11, 18–20, 24, 28, 30, 49, 54, 86, 106, 111, 116, 118, 123, 137, 139, 142, 144, 159, 170

Lynch syndrome, 8

M

Mahtani (doctor), 61, 97, 180

MammaPrint, 5, 45, 103

mammograms, 38, 49, 55–56, 80, 108, 133, 157, 160, 169–70

Margaret Lynn, 159–60

Marlene, 106–8, 132

mastectomy, 4–5, 35–36, 39, 47, 49–50, 62, 73–74, 97, 100, 134, 147, 151, 153, 161, 168, 170

   bilateral, 11, 24, 28, 54, 56, 76, 124, 134, 157–58

MBC, 1, 4–5, 23, 122

MBC (metastatic breast cancer), iii, 1–7, 9–11, 13, 15, 17, 19, 22–23, 25, 29, 31, 33–35, 37, 39, 42–43, 46–49, 51, 54–55, 57–65, 67–71, 73, 77, 79–81, 83, 85–87, 89, 92–97, 101, 103–7, 109, 111–13, 116–17, 119, 122–23, 125, 127–29, 131–33, 135, 137–39, 141–43, 145, 147, 150–51, 153, 155, 157, 159, 161, 169, 174–75

diagnosis of, 65, 79, 122–23, 138, 174

MD Anderson Cancer Center, 1, 4, 32, 48, 153, 178

melanoma, 19

memantine, 129–30

metastases, 4, 23, 34–35, 39, 48, 54, 60, 107, 116, 128, 134–35

bone, 6, 42, 48, 55, 64, 67, 76–77, 79, 106, 111, 116–17, 123

   brain, 105, 128–30, 132, 137–38, 142–43, 147, 165

   liver, 84, 131–32

   ovarian, 34, 43–44

Mildred, 59, 61, 73–74, 80

Moffitt Cancer Center, 143–44

MRI (magnetic resonance imaging), 73, 106, 111, 124, 137, 144, 157–58

MSFR (median survival from first relapse), 3–4

mutations, 8, 65, 68, 86, 107–8, 151

   genetic, 7–8, 64–65

   somatic, 68, 86

N

Navelbine, 47, 50, 54, 68, 76, 85, 94, 104, 123, 137, 163

NCI (National Cancer Institute), 164–65, 177

NED (no evidence disease), 47, 73, 125–26

NED (no evidence of disease), stage IV, 22, 48, 59, 159

neratinib, 7, 100, 104, 128–29, 138, 143

next-generation sequencing, 68, 107–8

nurses, 36, 40, 56–57, 77, 81, 97, 112, 120, 134–35, 144

O

oncologist, 5, 107

   medical, 5, 62, 153, 175

   radiation, 5, 51, 144, 153, 175, 178

osteoporosis, 33, 38

ovaries, 13, 19–20, 28, 34, 36, 38, 42–43, 45, 54–55, 84, 87, 102

Made in the USA
Las Vegas, NV
09 November 2023

80543099R00116